Nutritional Intelligence

Nutritional Intelligence

The Answer to Bulimia, Overeating, and Obesity

Evangelos Zoumbaneas

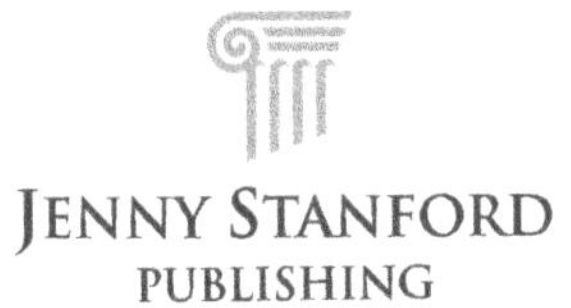
JENNY STANFORD
PUBLISHING

Published by

Jenny Stanford Publishing Pte. Ltd.
101 Thomson Road
#06-01, United Square
Singapore 307591

Email: editorial@jennystanford.com
Web: www.jennystanford.com

British Library Cataloguing-in-Publication Data
A catalogue record for this book is available from the British Library.

Nutritional Intelligence: The Answer to Bulimia, Overeating, and Obesity

Translated by Dimitra Lioliou, Spyridon Tsevas
English revision: Vicky Skarvatsopoulou
Previous edition's cover and book design: Eleni Achilleopoulou (PrintingSolutions.gr)
Cover image: ©Rawpixel

ISBN 978-981-5129-74-8 (Hardcover)
ISBN 978-981-5129-73-1 (Paperback)
ISBN 978-1-003-65188-8 (eBook)

To Agisilaos, Maya-Maria and little Helen
with the promise to make up for the time
I have stolen from our games

Contents

Introduction

As we look forward to the refreshed edition of the book *Nutritional Intelligence*, reflecting on the past decade, I had never imagined so many excellent health professionals would stand out from the "Master Practitioner in Eating Disorders" training course of the Centre for Education and Treatment of Eating Disorders (CETED).

Each of the trainers had not imagined that we would, through the inspiring training of **Deanne Jade** from the **National Centre for Eating Disorders** (NCFED) in Great Britain (eating-disorders.org.uk/) (the Professional Training Courses in Eating Disorders & Obesity), not only convey some knowledge on eating disorders—which anyone could get by reading relative books or watching an e-learning course—but also create new teachers, talented therapists, charismatic authors and bright professionals who stand out for their ethics and love for the people who desperately need their help.

Everyone's starting point was *Nutritional Intelligence*, a landmark book, which was the key motivation for, primarily, personal change in each of them and, the transformation of this change into new knowledge, in the form of inspiring books and catalytic therapeutic skills. I am thrilled by the mere thought of the many more inspiring and charismatic members the CETED family can add to its ranks in the future.

Though I am sure that the company of my charismatic collaborators will always have room for new skills, more inspiration and wonderful surprises for all people with natural talent, who want to be a part of the CETED family. I admire these bright brains; I thrive in the notion that I was responsible for giving all these individuals the chance to come out through this course. I am grateful for all I have already offered, and all I will be able to give in the future because the graduates' expression and sensitivity have come to touch and soothe my soul. Special thanks to my teachers Deanne Jade, principal of NCFED, and nutritionist Jane Nodder, my closest associates psychologist Dr Margarita-Aggeliki Schina and nutritionist Mrs Ioanna Kontele, as well as all the trainers of CETED in Greece.

After all, as we the trainers of CETED say, the only scenario for the treatment of eating disorders is that...

"There is no other scenario!"

Evangelos Zoumbaneas
Clinical Dietitian-Nutritionist
Master Practitioner on Eating Disorders
Director of the Centre for Education and Treatment
of Eating Disorders, Greece (www.keadd.gr)

Chapter 1

"Working" with Bulimia

Bulimia mainly affects talented people who had never been able to unfold their talent.

1.1 "Forwarding" Bulimia...

The maximum sustainability of a hypocaloric nutrition schedule for a person suffering from an eating disorder is, on average, two months. The next step is the interruption of the diet and rapid return to the weight level the individual was at when first going on this diet, perhaps even exceeding it. Through this process, every two months the person interrupts the diet and goes on to a new "magic" weight loss method.

This has nothing to do with lack of willpower but the disruption of the body's natural defence mechanisms. It is irrelevant to the fact that two months after starting, there probably wasn't enough motivation for further weight-loss, but it is owed to the loss of the magic keys that will lock the "beast" of bulimia back to its cage. It will always be there, every single day and hour. Every time a meal is lost or every time the person wants to eat more than what is recommended in their diet plan, it lurks, waiting for the first moment of weakness to devour them.

If bulimia is treated thoughtlessly, if a person doesn't learn how to deal with it, if they don't understand the mechanisms and techniques required to be able to tame it, then this beast is probably going to grow old with them. The person ends up wasting their life

Nutritional Intelligence: The Answer to Bulimia, Overeating, and Obesity
Evangelos Zoumbaneas

ISBN 978-981-5129-74-8 (Hardcover), 978-981-5129-73-1 (Paperback), 978-1-003-65188-8 (eBook)
www.jennystanford.com

being on unsuccessful diets. The more diets one follows, the more the beast of bulimia is strengthened until it dominates and forces the person to compromise and live with their obesity.

And yet, bulimia can be treated. It takes brains, not brawn. In order to defeat it, you need to get to know it. To recognise its weaknesses, learn how to tame it, find its vulnerable spots, and plan how to face it in a "hand to hand" combat. The solutions lie inside you and the secret of winning is to learn to recognise which mechanisms bulimia itself plays on to break your defences.

The first step to success is to begin anew having reinforced the physiological defence mechanisms your body already possesses. Knowledge is power. By acquiring knowledge, you will gradually manage to outpower your rival and eventually beat it. It is essential you manage to be thin at some point, but you must also be strong.

Let's venture on a trip together now, in search of the hidden treasure: to collect the keys that will help you tame bulimia and open the chest that hides the lost treasure of charm.

1.2 Introduction

1.2.1 The Criteria for Bulimia

> *"It is evening, and I have just finished my errands. This is the only time I can devote to myself, stay alone, relax. A short while ago, I had a salad for dinner, since I'm on a diet... again. Unfortunately, the idea of some chocolate hidden in the cupboard is spinning around my head. I shouldn't eat it... I shouldn't break my diet... but I want it... I won't rest if I don't eat a little chocolate... I will eat just a little bit and then stop... A little chocolate... A few biscuits ... some cheese with a slice of bread, Ah! There is also a piece of feta cheese pie in the oven... and some leftovers from yesterday... let's eat the rest of the chocolate; besides, I have already broken the diet! I'm such a pig! I couldn't manage to keep the diet again. I've ruined it all! I'm fat and useless!"*

Does this description perhaps remind you of parts of your life? I personally believe that few people have avoided going through a similar thought process altogether. These could be Eva's, the girl next door, words soon after an uncontrolled bulimic episode. Before examining how to deal with bulimia, let's focus on the two common eating disorders relating to binge eating.

My colleague Ioanna Kontele refers to them below in a comprehensible way, as published in the 20th issue of "Diatrofi

Health & Wellness" magazine by the "Diatrofi" scientific team of nutritionists.

When the cycle of binge eating and the following guilt is prevalent for a considerable time period, we are facing a widespread condition called *binge eating disorder.* Suppose these episodes are also accompanied by compensatory behaviours, such as vomiting, overexercising, use of laxatives and diuretics, or fasting, we are up against a dangerous eating disorder called *bulimia nervosa*. The common denominators, as found in the tables of criteria are binge-eating episodes, loss of control, and subsequent guilt.

Criteria Of Binge Eating Disorder (Dsm-5)	**Criteria Of Bulimia Nervosa (Dsm-5)**
1. Recurring binge-eating episodes during which a large amount of food is consumed in a short time.	1. Multiple binge-eating episodes when a large amount of food is consumed in a short time.
2. During those episodes, there is an intense loss of control: the person feels that they cannot stop eating.	2. During those episodes there is an intense loss of control, the person feels that they cannot stop eating.
3. During those episodes, at least three of the following steps occur: - The person eats faster than regular. - The person eats until they feel discomfort. - The person consumes large quantities of food without feeling hungry. - The person eats privately because they feel embarrassed. - The person feels disgusted of themselves and a great deal of guilt. - There is intense discomfort after the binge-eating episode.	3. Repeated inappropriate compensatory behaviour (self-provoked vomiting, use of laxatives and diuretics, fast, over exercising). 4. The binge-eating episodes take place on average 2 times per week for 3 months. 5. Self-evaluation is extremely affected by the weight and the shape of the body.
4. Binge-eating episodes take place on average 2 times per week for 6 months	
5. Methods of purging or weight control are not used (vomiting, overexercising, etc.)	

There are few studies that have investigated the occurrence of binge eating disorder among the population. Evidence shows that 3% of the population matches the criteria for binge eating disorder. In obese people this percentage is 8%, while the rate is even higher in people with diabetes mellitus type 2. Among the people who consult a specialist to lose weight, 30% cover all the disorder criteria. Even though the general population percentage is not very high, there are many people with atypical forms of the disorder, which means that they cover some of the criteria; for instance, binge-eating episodes are not very intense, but the person still feels a lot of guilts. These people experience the same psychological stress, and need help as well.

Bulimia nervosa seems to appear in 1-1.4% of the population, but the atypical forms where e.g., these behaviours occur less frequently, add even more to that number. Also, it should be considered that people who participate in studies don't usually mention that they vomit, use laxatives or excessive exercising for fear of embarrassment and as a result, the possibility of bulimia nervosa in such cases escapes documentation.

1.3 Factors for the Development of Bulimia and Binge Eating

1.3.1 Reflecting on a Real-Life Case

The incident we will examine is a clinical case of a "yo-yo" diet with characteristics of emotional disorder. Using the term "yo-yo" diet, we mean to describe all those numerous cases of people whose weight has gone up and down so often, just like the cylinder of the child's toy, rhythmically wrapped and unwrapped on a thread. A thread that breaks due to the constant wrapping, shattering the self-confidence and self-respect of millions of people who are consumed in a failed diet throughout almost their entire life. A life lost in more and more extreme diets and harrowing techniques. As a result, these people become vulnerable to every form of manipulation because of their pain and victims of malicious behaviours whose sole purpose is the desperate victims' financial drainage through the informal economy and the "slimming cartels".

The incident which we will investigate is one of the most classic examples of a woman who from adolescence till now– in her 50s – has been consumed in diets and techniques of every form, with the sole outcome of gaining weight shortly after every diet but also the constant accumulation of psychological and emotional pressure.

Firstly, to be able to understand her psychological condition and the reasons that led her to increased levels of obesity, the related cultural factors and their effect to body image and self-respect will be analysed.

In other words, we will try to walk in her shoes, to follow her path in clear and simple steps up to the present day by thumbing through every page, reading all the critical stages of her life that were milestones in the repetitive relapses of the diet. Also, a more specialised analysis will be performed, regarding the emotional disorder and "how every emotion can affect the way this woman eats." Furthermore, the family factors and how some family members play an essential role in the evolution of the disorder will be examined. Her psychological development is also worth mentioning, especially during adolescence, since the constant weight fluctuation of this individual started during adolescence. For many psychologists, this particular method constitutes "a free flight to maturity," which is clearly affected by the winds that happen to be blowing each moment.

To understand and elicit all the information that will be presented next, five meetings with Evi were deemed necessary, whose case was the reason for writing this book. Through those sessions and through the collaboration with psychologist Androula Ilia, the objectives, interventions, assumptions, difficulties, this woman's realisations, as well as the results of the meetings will unravel.

1.3.2 Why Was This Case Chosen?

There are plenty of reasons why I opted to examine this specific case. Taking into consideration that this woman has lost a significant amount of weight (at least 2 times, she has lost 20-30 kilos which she always gained back) we explained to her that it was time she had seen things from a perspective beyond dieting and that she had to start realising that the reasons why she wasn't able to maintain the desired weight were much deeper. The only thing she had in mind until then was that she felt unable and that her primary problem was lack of self-control. Due to the experience she had gained from all previews diets, she already knew enough about nutrition. However, she couldn't control it. Often (at least two to three times per week), she lost control and had bulimic episodes (cravings). This fact caused us to look for and examine the causes of this failure. How was such a knowledgeable woman unable to control her nutrition? Why did so much effort, in cooperation with a nutritionist, always go to waste? At the same time, we had to follow another procedure of reasoning and knowledge regarding what this woman was able to do from then on.

1.3.3 Cultural Factors

It is vital that the case must start with an examination of the cultural factors. This woman lived in Greece, and particularly Athens, in a traditional, but at the same time, modern environment. It is this environment that caused internal conflicts since she had been raised in a family that followed traditional values. For many years, she had been living as a modern woman - alone and independent. Contemporary lifestyle demanded that this young woman be independent and comply with the requirements of contemporary society. Traditionally, the role of a woman in the Greek family is to serve everyone's needs, to please them all and as a result, lose contact with her personal needs. This situation puts the person under enormous psychological pressure, simultaneously trying to meet the contemporary female standards, yet never managing to do so because, within the family context, she is called to also serve other roles that contradict her desires. This situation affected most women who lived not only in Athens but also in all big cities whose social norms lie between contemporary and traditional, mixing values and principles. This phenomenon is also common in villages and smaller towns, where generally there is a tendency of young people fleeing to bigger, and thus more modernised, cities.

1.3.4 Emotional or Mood Disorder

It is very important to focus on this woman's emotional disorder since it is a frequent but at the same time complicated case. Its difficulty lies in the fact that the dietician can't fight a situation like that through cognitive methods, that is by using knowledge and experience: "Yes, I know that what I do is bad, so I will stop it". An emotional disorder, along with Greek culture, cannot be soothed through simple procedures because the emotions loom. If the emotions aren't appeased, if they don't find answers and ways out, however much she may know, whatever anyone knows, there's no way the problems caused by the emotional disorder can be dealt with. For this reason, we often come across people like Evi who despite being an educated and informed person, at the same time she "sabotages," all this cognitive part and gets carried away in tactics that knowingly harm her but which she cannot in any way control.

1.3.5 The Role of Stress

At the same time, we will examine the role of stress in emotional disorders, which is especially important, since it is an undifferentiated emotional state in which the person feels tension without knowing what exactly is taking place. When stress is particularly intense due to any reason, a person is not capable of following any form of diet. We could say that under the influence of stress, a person cannot take care of himself or do anything beneficial for himself, even if they know what they want or should do. So, we consider it as a significant setback in achieving the aim. It is also significant we go further into the factors that cause stress for the individual, such as cultural (e.g., the fact that she has to be slim 'till summer), interfamilial (e.g., disease in the family), work, etc., to see to what degree she is ready to make an effort. The evaluation of stress through specific tests is considered necessary so that the patient's readiness to begin a diet in the specific phase of their life is determined. (See p. 34).

1.3.6 Depression

We gradually need to focus on the emotional situations since this woman could be suffering from a type of depression that might be pathogenic. Depression is not necessarily endogenous, accompanied by a sickness and requiring medication. We need to understand where the depression comes form, what the sorrow that the person feels is, in other words, to investigate the grief and its origin. It may derive, for instance, from failures in her life or the fact that she is not happy with her body. Many women, trying to be the way society wants them to be, experience personal failures that cause them sadness, which we cannot easily define as endogenous or attribute to other causes.

1.3.7 Difficulty in Solving Conflicts and Inability to Deal with Anger

Another critical emotional situation is difficulty in solving conflicts. This is a fundamental issue, especially in people who, in a social context, seem easy-going, but at the same time have trouble finding solutions for conflicts and getting results through this. These people usually swallow their anger and other emotions e.g., happiness, because there is a cultural prejudice in Greece that if you express your happiness to people, they will jinx it, you and something terrible will happen to you.

1.3.8 Emotional and Existential Void

These people also intensely experience emotional void. The emotion of emptiness is prevalent in obesity, and it is very frequent, during therapy, to feel that the patient or the client never stops, gets satiated or is unable to stop. The therapist needs to keep giving, caring for and supporting without cease. Sometimes, he gets exhausted (professional burn out). This gap needs to be covered by the client who should realise that if they don't put an end to this downfall themselves, they will not be treated. At a physical level, the message of satiation may be expressed through serotonin or other messages released by the body and lead to a pause of food intake (extensively analysed in Part A of Chapter 2). But there is also the psychological hunger which could be interpreted in many ways, such as the fact that the person wasn't given adequate nourishment during childhood or didn't receive all the emotional support that they should have during the first year of their life, or that all these unreceived emotions have been replaced by material goods. The person thus learned how to feed on the possession of material goods and not emotions.

There is still one void, this time an existential one. It concerns people who are existentially lost and as they are unaware of what can satiate them, they keep looking to fill this void, food being the most readily available solution. It could also be alcohol or drugs for some others, and it is common for eating disorders to be treated the same way as alcoholism or rehabilitation from drug addiction.

1.3.9 Social Phobia

The term refers to the person's fear of being subjected to attention as well as criticism by their environment.

Another matter comes in the form of the phobic person - he who is afraid to externalise. If we look at fat as a shield, as a means of defence, the obese person, having the shell of obesity around them, is afraid to go out without their protection. If this defence is not replaced by internal way of self-protection, they won't be able to lower it. This could explain the fluctuation of weight because if the person loses their defence unprepared, or having found ways to protect themselves and resist, they will soon gain back all the weight since it is their shield. It is proven that if inner work is not done, the person will relapse very quickly and soon go back to where they started bearing more physical and psychological weight.

1.3.10 Guilt

Guilt is also a significant factor. It is a situation which could be interpreted as shame in Greece. The person may feel ashamed for several things (e.g., his/her gender), therefore using food as self-punishment. The way food is used in western culture, it is connected to punishment. The subconscious conveys the message: "Since I'm not the way I am supposed to be, I must be punished." This is why, during relapses, we consider essential to understand why the person is punished. An aim of the therapeutic procedure is to hinder self-destruction and reduce its impact.

1.3.11 Difficulties during Adolescence

Another critical issue is the fact that many nutritional difficulties begin during adolescence. These disorders are also related to gender related disorders. If during adolescence, when the person chooses their sexual orientation, they blame themselves, get confused with, or scared of their own existence as a woman or a man, food provides a way out of dealing with what he or she is, or in fact what nature obliges them to be. This is the definition of "flight", which means the person backs away from dealing with what is happening to them. He picks a way out, which eventually is also destructive.

1.3.12 Self-Esteem

Self-esteem is not about the achievements of a person. Obese people with emotional disorders have hurt their self-esteem by gaining and losing weight. They believe that they haven't achieved anything significant as their physical appearance has monopolised their self-image and they feel socially rejected. This is the trap when it comes to self-esteem and the solution is to gradually separate their physical appearance from their image of self and begin seeing themselves in a broader perspective, not only as a physical presence. Apart from their body, the person should also note their achievements so as to rely on them and subsequently work on their body.

1.3.13 Loneliness

Another crucial element is loneliness. In big cities like Athens, it is predominant among women and men and is frequently coped with food. When the person is alone in their apartment, food will cover their loneliness, which is connected to social failure, existential loneliness and many more emotions which the person cannot face.

1.3.14 Expression of Emotions

Another issue comes with unexpressed emotions since those people are not trained to understand how they feel and think food is the primary solution as it is cheap and easily obtainable. It is usual for many people to lack in ability to recognise the particular emotion that drives them to impulsive actions.

1.3.15 Emotional Intelligence

In this part, we will talk about the Emotional Intelligence Quality index, since a lot of people have a very low emotional intelligence, which means that they are not patient and don't wish to wait, thus their brain learns to act very fast to cover the needs at a primary level and through a primitive way – a defence mechanism against the dangers of surviving in a hostile environment. In more emotionally advanced people who can wait, the brain simultaneously creates broader networks, interconnections, new neurons, and, at that time, deepens and processes what is happening, why it is happening, why it has to react in one way or another. Thus, patience grows, maturity evolves, and therefore emotional intelligence is cultivated. So next time the person is about to deal with a similar situation, it will be more empowered. They will have created a sturdier resistance. Every time they control even a few of these impulsive reactions, they will feel more resilient against any challenge. A good exercise for those people is waiting, e.g., wait for 5 minutes, put down the fork, chew slowly, get some fresh air for 2 minutes, and call somebody to talk to, take ten deep breaths. This way, the person increases his resistance. A classic example that works in people with emotional disorders is the Stanford candy experiment by Walter Michel, professor at the University of Stanford, involving kids and candies where a dilemma was presented to a child: "Do you want a marshmallow now or two marshmallows but wait for a little while?" Following the experiment's study, several years later upon evaluation of the children who had chosen to receive two candies by waiting for a little, it was found that they had made better life choices later as teenagers. In contrast, the children who did not wait at all had difficulties during adolescence. This means that they were significantly connected with their Emotional Intelligence Quality index in whatever choices they made in their life.

1.3.16 Personalisation

Finally, we consider very important to clarify that every case is unique. We shouldn't believe that the same assumptions and interventions must be made because of the existence of corresponding cases. This particular case is unique, and this will be the principle on which we will base our future work. Evi's case will be the motive to understand that obese and bulimic people's lives are connected to a series of unsuccessful diets. These people need a different approach, outside the framework of a proper sub-caloric nutrition which undoubtedly is one of the determinants in the treatment of obesity, but certainly not the only one.

1.3.17 The Background of the Diet and Weight Fluctuation "Lifeline"

Before we proceed to the description and analysis of the sessions, we will present the different stages of this case's weight fluctuation and the person's weight development. Evi's "Lifeline" begins making a small reference to her body weight during childhood. Starting from the first incident which was the cause for her to start eating uncontrollably but also the first day she went on a diet during adolescence; we observe that the weight variation line changes shockingly until today. The determining points of every unsuccessful diet which led her to her biggest weight are described step by step. The "Lifeline" is one of the first, and defining, information received while taking the patient's history. It is about an essential procedure during which the person in front of us starts unravelling the tangle of their memories. This process is necessary to elicit the information that will help us later during the treatment process. It will be the first revelation on how the patient got here. In the history and the diagram below, all the important facts that affected the start or the end of a diet are presented one by one, while monitoring the exact bodyweight in each period in combination with the age and the corresponding life period. The "Lifeline" procedure is the powerful weapon of both the patient and the therapist, often rocking long-established situations which find the opportunity to dislodge and reveal the secrets and issues below, for the latter to then be processed. Evi's example, as well as the deriving conclusions are shocking. Before we move on, it's worth taking a careful look at the crazy race of weight gain and loss in the case examined below.

1.3.18 Case Study: Evi's Weight Fluctuation

- March 1963: **date of birth**, body weight: **3.250 kilos**.
- **14 years old**, height: 150 cm, weight: **40 kilos**. As far as she can remember herself in the early stages of puberty, she was a normal kid with nutritional problems.
- **15 years old**, height: 155 cm, weight: **55 kilos**. High school starts.
- **17 years old**, height: 158 cm, weight: **60 kilos**. This is the age of her first heartbreak, and the first time she starts gaining weight.
- **18 years old**, height: 158 cm, weight: **65 kilos**. In September 1981, she starts studying journalism, and, in the same period, she works in a newspaper. The work environment is quite bad, with many difficulties, and this situation causes very low self-esteem.
- **20 years old**, weight: **90 kilos**. In October 1983, she graduates from university, stops working in the newspaper and gets a job as a public officer. This situation makes her feel secure and safe. At the same time, she gets into a new relationship with a very slim guy who encourages her to go on a diet.
- **22 years old**, weight: **65 kilos**. Two years later, she has managed to lose weight in her own way and with her boyfriend's support. It is a good period for her.
- **26 years old**, weight: **64.6 kilos**. February 5, 1989. She breaks up with her boyfriend, so that is a bad period in her life. She is afraid that she will start gaining weight, so she decides to ask for help from a weight loss institute. On March 5, 1989, they persuade her to undergo treatment to lose 10 kilos in 10 weeks. So, after she has signed a contract, she goes on an extreme diet. She struggles due to the intense physical fatigue caused by the lack of essential nutrients.
- **26 years old**, on 8th August, weight: **59 kilos**. That means it took 5 months of collaboration with the institute to get to this weight (almost 5.6 kilos in 20 weeks, contrary to the promised 10 pounds in 10 weeks). She feels disappointed and starts gaining weight again.

- **27 years old**, weight: **75 kilos**. She starts a new diet unsupervised by a specialist. She takes up physical activity.
- **28 years old**, weight: **58 kilos**. After 14 months, she manages to reach a weight of 58 kilos. She gets into a new relationship with a 42-year-old man (14 years older than her). The main characteristics are that he is an obese man weighing over 120 kilos. Every night, his only entertainment is going out to good restaurants.
- **29 years old**, weight: **80 kilos**. At this age, her relationship with the older man ends and this is another challenging time in her life. Due to the significant amount of fatty food, she consumed every night, she already weighed 80 kilos. Then, she goes on a new diet without supervision.
- **31 years old**, weight: **65 - 70 kilos**. Two years later, she manages to lose weight in her own way and with her boyfriend's support. For 6 months, her weight ranges from 65 to 70 kilos. At this time the family finds out about the rare disease of her brother's 1-month-old child. This is too much for her and she spends a week ingesting nothing but water. After this week, she starts eating again. The next 4 years will be challenging. She is alone without any support from her friends. Additionally, she carries the entire psychological burden of supporting her whole family.
- **35 years old**, weight: **96 kilos**. After 4 years, she weighs 96 kilos for the first time and seems unable of comprehending how this has happened. She has wasted all her energy and thoughts supporting her family and she has abandoned herself. She realises her problem with weight when she falls in love with a man. She gets into a relationship with him and he supports her with her diet. He is a very skinny man; she really tries to please him and she is always agreeable with him.
- **36 years old**, weight: **85 kilos**. At this age, her relationship with her boyfriend ends and this is another tough time in her life. After that, she starts eating again.
- **36.5 years old**, weight: **96 pounds**. After a 6-month period of over-eating, she weighs a lot. For the next 6 months, her weight remains stable.

- **37 years old**, weight: **95 kilos**. She starts a new diet by herself. She also takes up physical activity.
- **38 years old**, weight: **74.3 kilos**. Sixteen months later, she manages to lose weight in her own way. She realises that it is challenging to continue trying by herself, and she decides to ask for help from a professional dietitian. He provides her with a healthy weekly nutritional program, and he suggests that she take up walking. Coincidentally, the date of commencement of the diet is on September 11, 2001, just before the moment the World Trade Centre collapsed in New York.
- **39 years old,** weight: **67 kilos**. On September 9, after 12 months, with the dietitian's weekly help, she manages to lose much weight. She feels very excited because this change has happened without following a strict diet but through a proper meal plan and light physical activity. Her dietitian suggests that she continue her appointments once a month. Furthermore, he suggests she buy new clothes, visit a psychologist and talk about her new body image. She follows none of his advice and stops consulting with him.
- **40 years old**, weight: **76.8 kilos**. February 27, 2003. After 16 months, she Has gained 10 kilos. She has spent all her energy and thoughts on her family for another time, so she has abandoned herself again. She wants to go back to her dietitian, but she feels guilty and ashamed. She finds the courage to do it when she falls in love with a man. She does not enter a relationship with him but goes on a new diet because she wants to impress him.
- **41 years old**, weight: **70.8 kilos**. May 14, 2003. After 3 months, she weighs but 6 kilos less. She feels really disappointed, mainly because she believes that she cannot do anything of what the dietitian says. Her dietitian explains that her body is exhausted from all the efforts to lose weight, so she needs to be patient. At the same time, the man with whom she has fallen in love marries another woman, which is the final blow for her.
- **41 years old**, weight: **91 kilos**. January 14, 2004. After 8 months, she gains 20.2 kilos. She returns to her dietitian for

another try. Her weight has caused problems to her knees. The doctor tries to convince her of the importance of losing weight in a bad manner, telling her that she has to lose 45 pounds immediately. This behaviour makes her furious, and for a long time, she goes off her diet.

- **42 years old**, weight: **82.5 kilos**. July 21st, 2004. She manages to lose 8.5 kilos. Due to being overweight, she still has problems with her knees, which is why she cannot exercise. During the same period, her mother needs to undergo surgery due to breast cancer. Therefore, under all this pressure, she reacts in the only way she knows: She starts eating again and goes off her diet. After several months, she will spend an extended period in hospitals due to her father's heart failure.
- **44 years old** weight: **96 kilos**. 14th March 2006 Most of her family's problems are under control. She returns to her dietitian, and at this point, they start the consultative meeting with the psychologist as described below.
- **44 years** old weight: **92 kilos**. May 20th, 2006 Two months later, she loses 4 kilos effortlessly. She already knows what proper nutritional serves its purpose, so she doesn't have any problem following a healthy meal plan. After managing her eating disorders in cooperation with her dietitian and psychologist, she reports that she feels much better. Since she has got away from her guilt, she starts comprehending her needs. She starts expressing her anger and setting limits with the people of her environment. Additionally, she has managed to set a limit to the quantity of food that she used to eat and from a love-hate relationship, now she actually enjoys every meal. She believes it is her duty to protect herself and has realised that it is often necessary to ask for help from other people whom she trusts and have the knowledge and will to guide and help her.

In the diagram, the vertical column shows the weight fluctuation from the (theoretical) ideal weight of 65 pounds respectively to age. It appears in the horizontal column. Within the text framework, the key factors that have affected Evi's life and the variation of her weight are mentioned briefly.

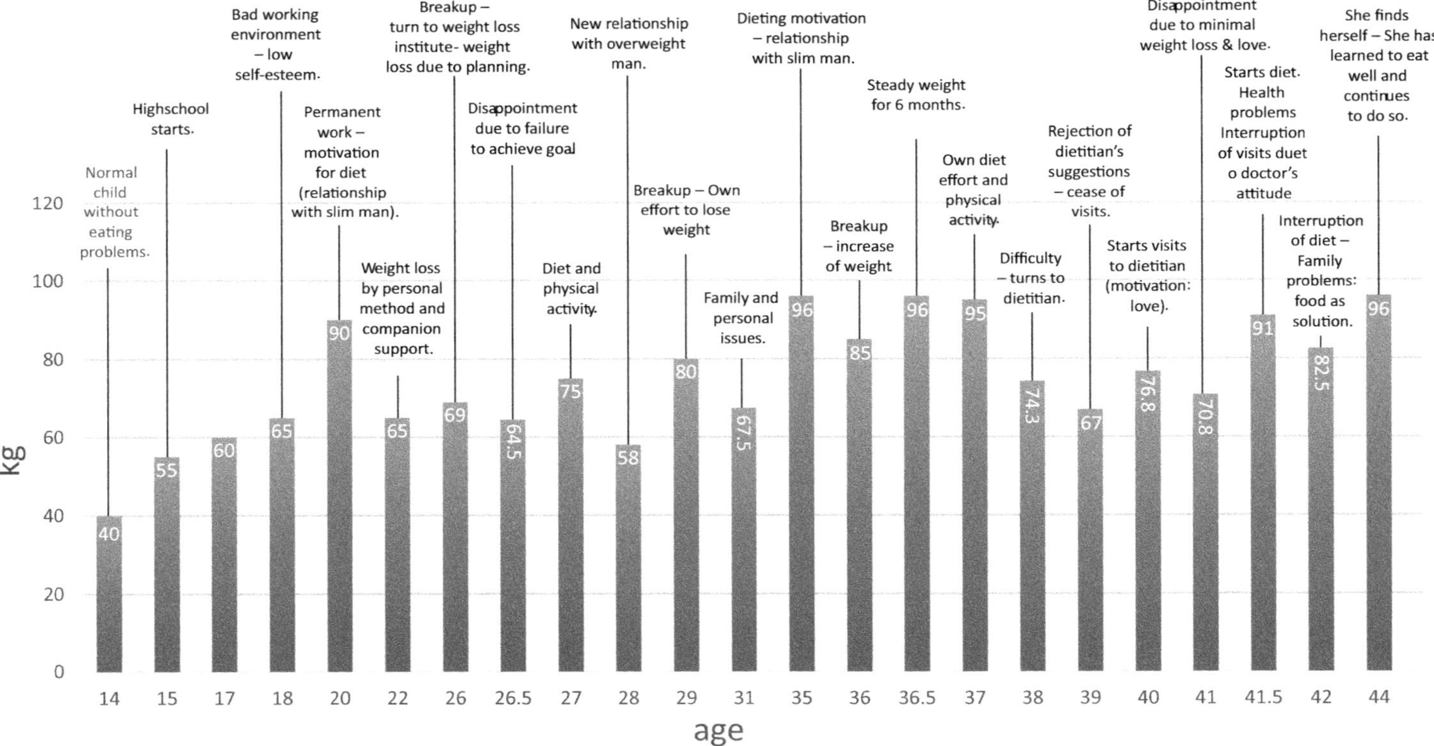
Normal child without eating problems.
Highschool starts.
Bad working environment – low self-esteem.
Permanent work – motivation for diet (relationship with slim man).
Weight loss by personal method and companion support.
Breakup – turn to weight loss institute- weight loss due to planning.
Disappointment due to failure to achieve goal
Diet and physical activity.
New relationship with overweight man.
Breakup – Own effort to lose weight
Family and personal issues.
Dieting motivation – relationship with slim man.
Breakup – increase of weight
Steady weight for 6 months.
Own diet effort and physical activity.
Difficulty – turns to dietitian.
Rejection of dietitian's suggestions – cease of visits.
Starts visits to dietitian (motivation: love).
Disappointment due to minimal weight loss & love.
Starts diet. Health problems Interruption of visits duet o doctor's attitude
Interruption of diet – Family problems: food as solution.
She finds herself – She has learned to eat well and continues to do so.
40
55
60
65
90
65
69
64.5
75
58
80
67.5
96
85
96
95
74.3
67
76.8
70.8
91
82.5
96
kg
0
20
40
60
80
100
120
14
15
17
18
20
22
26
26.5
27
28
29
31
35
36
36.5
37
38
39
40
41
41.5
42
44
age

1.4 Psychological and Nutritional Approach for Bulimia and Binge Eating: Meeting/Sessions

Following are the notes from Evi's five consultation sessions with the psychologist and dietitian.

1.4.1 First Meeting: March 14, 2006

The first meeting aims to provide an opportunity to get to know the person, we try to take a fist look into the causes and situations that lead to the bulimic episodes and give a complete explanation of how food and not dieting can help limit the bulimic episodes.

1.4.1.1 History

Evi is 44 years old and works as a civil servant. She does not have much free time, lives alone, but at the same time, she often visits her parents and takes care of them. She is the second child of the family. Her family is facing many health issues. Her father has chronic heart failure, her mother has undergone mastectomy, and her brother has a child with a severe health condition. She has taken on the role of supporting the members of her family and feels a lot of pain and anxiety for their lives and what goes on in her family. What is constantly being said to her is that her needs are secondary, meaning that since her family members deal with more serious problems, she ought to avoid complaining and expressing negativity. This, consequently, results in her feeling depressed, pressed and therefore, she stays at home and has bulimic episodes. She didn't have weight problems at an early age, despite never considering herself as thin. During adolescence she started gaining weight, and at the age of 20 she was already overweight. As she mentions, she started consuming extreme quantities of food after a heartbreak at the age of 17. Since the age of 20 she was frequently on a diet and her weight fluctuations reached up to 30 kilos. OVER the last four years, she has put on 30 kilos over the weight limit considered normal for her, which ranges from 58 to 65 kilos according to the Body Mass Index (BMI) (height: 160cm.). Her mother underwent a mastectomy during those four years, which spawned several fears in her. During this period, her duty was to support her mother, and food, as she mentions, was a shelter or a way out for her. Her mother's health problem started soon after her last successful effort. She lost several kilos for the 2nd time in collaboration with a dietitian. Since her mother's health problem appeared, she had gained all the weight she had lost, in an almost respective period, and has kept gaining weight until today, reaching 90 kilos. Her major weight fluctuations create a feeling of futility in her. "Yo-yo" diets have substantially reduced her self-esteem resulting in her not knowing who to rely on and where to find support. We also talk about the difficulty in expressing her anger. She describes to us that she goes home and eats uncontrollably when she gets angry with somebody. As she points out, upon returning home around 10 pm the first thing she does is order great amounts of food and keep eating almost as if being hypnotized.

1.4.1.2 Intervention on the subject of anger and feelings

Through this intervention, we will help her focus on how to express her feelings and thoughts. What she has done so far is to react to others and not assert herself or express her thoughts. Reacting this way, she distances herself and withdraws. In the first session, she has already started talking about how she is burdened with problems and responsibilities and starts to unravel her thoughts and feelings. Through the Socratic Method, by asking questions and letting her find the answers, she recalls data from her memory. She strengthens her position and starts expressing her feelings. She starts realising that she has the right to feel anger and demand what she needs, and we try to support her in this as much as possible. Through consultative support, we train her to learn more about herself and identify her anger and how she is drawn, because of the anger, into actions that she later regrets. She has become more skilful in expressing her anger while at the same time, we support her in her effort to go out and do it. It is important to note that she has stated that it is forbidden to express herself intensively within her professional framework. She has an explicit mandate by her supervisor not to cause any tensions, always keep her voice down, and cover up everything that is going on. Through discussion, we try to enhance her self-esteem so that she can express herself. Since she is a 44-year-old woman with 24 years of work experience, she can rely on her knowledge and express herself, express what she feels, thinks, and goes through.

1.4.1.3 Intervention on the matter of binge-eating

During the 1st meeting, through several discussions, we came to understand how she eats. What difficulties she faces, where she loses control and which the difficult hours are. As we said before, she has mentioned that the episodes take place when she returns home at 10 o'clock. She described to us that the binge-eating episodes are her refuge, acting as a safety net. It is the only time she has for herself, while all other times are for everybody. But the next morning, she feels terrible. At this point, we talked about any alternatives and the help that her friends can offer. She mentioned that she does not find any support from the relationships with her friends, but, at the same time, through discussion, she gets to realise that this happens because she does not ask their help. She feels like nobody is capable of shouldering her burden. The positive thing is that when she is with people with whom she can communicate pleasantly, she does not think about food, e.g., when she is in the painting group where she feels comfortable and can express herself. On the contrary, in the choir, where she does not relate with the other members and which she just attends because she likes the activity, there are moments when she thinks of food. She does not feel the same safety and warmth there. So, we suggested that, during the difficult times of the night, when she is overwhelmed by binge-eating episodes, she should call her friend or engage in some activity that would get her out of her routine. If she finds the power to do so, it will distract her from binge-eating episodes, then she will be able to use that power to cope with the difficult moments. To be able to make a correlation between her feelings and the binge-eating episodes, we have provided her with a form to keep track of the food she eats and at the same time, try to describe where she is when she does this, whom she is with, the degree of hunger she feels before starting the meal and what it feels like when eating. We explained, in simple terms, the mechanisms of serotonin and glucose in the body and how nutrition can influence a person's desire for food (these chapters are discussed in detail in Chapter 2).

1.4.1.4 The battle against bulimia is often lost before you even begin fighting it

We explained to her that the need for food can be triggered by psychological causes. Still, it may also be due to nutritional reasons and that the lack of valuable nutrients leads to a search for food intake. An excellent example we use to demonstrate this is the following: "Whether a human being is led to a binge-eating episodes depends on two factors. One has to do with nutritional, and the other with psychological factors. Imagine that our body plays a daily match, the result of which depends on the score of the two halves. Whether we win the first half depends on how well we are prepared on a nutritional level. If we ensure a good dietary result through the quality of our food as well as regular meals, then the first half is ours. Whether we lose the second half for psychological reasons, cannot be predicted at the start of the day. However, it is practically impossible that we'll lose the second half every day because of our mental state. But if we have already lost the first half because of our poor nutrition, then the game is lost before we even step foot on the field and unfortunately, the result of the defeat will be blamed on psychological reasons as a whole (vicious circle of bulimia - see table p. 114). So, let's win as many first halves as we can and then see how we will proceed afterwards. That is, even we have binge-eating episodes, let them happen after we have consumed everything that the body needs to receive proper care. And rest assured that the more appropriately combined nutrients you put into your body, the more you will gain the physio-organic strength to resist overeating. You will slowly begin reducing the caloric range of binge-eating episodes when you start eating correctly. For example, you can have a binge-eating episode of 2000 calories today, but tomorrow or the day after you will only need 1500 calories to stop eating. Next week you will need even less, and you will gradually begin reducing the frequency of these episodes. As your body gets more robust, and the more your skills and ability to understand what's going on inside you will be sharpened, the healthier you will be. That is why it is essential to know that we will first service your body as if it was a car, and then you will be able to drive it fast. We will first restore the balance of the appetite and satiety mechanisms and then move on to what's next".

This example has proved to always have a good effect on people with eating disorders. Malnourished people exist for a variety of reasons: they consume many calories due to poor nutrition, mainly due to eating food of high caloric value but very poor from a nutritional perspective. People often ask me how much weight they will lose per week or when they will have reached their goal, to which I answer with another question. "If you could imagine your body as a vehicle with a lot of damage: no brakes, no lights, no oils, with worn tires, it is like asking me, if you get on the highway, how fast you will get from New York to L.A.". The answer is "never". Even if you manage to get on the highway, you'll soon break down or get off the road on the first steep turn. That is why we will first repair the body, control the damage, and nourish all those mechanisms that will strengthen it and then see how we will move forward. The patient needs to understand the criticality of the situation at that moment, i.e., the first day he comes to us to start another diet. It is essential for them to realise through discussion and training that the body cannot function according to their expectations and a lot of talk is necessary about which of them are reasonable and to what degree. They must accept that first, proper preparation must be made for all those mechanisms to be able to support them and enable them to come closer to their goal.

Another key goal of her treatment is to destigmatise and create a better relationship with food. That is why she was told that at this point, we will not deal with her weight at all; there will be no weighing and we also asked her to put the weighing scales away at home, and avoid any weighing, even of the food she eats. We asked her, through the instructions given to her, to let herself free and try to listen to her inner needs, choosing what she wants to eat every time simply by trying to use the food combinations we have suggested to her and eat at regular intervals as described in detail in Chapter 3. At this point, we often use another example to help this in comprehending this method. "Many studies have shown that every time animals were force-fed to gain weight, to the point of doubling their initial weight, upon being allowed to be fed again by themselves they returned to their normal diet within a very short time. Subsequently, these animals instinctively reduced their food intake compared to what they had been eating in the past, and as a result returned to their normal weight after some time without any external intervention. The amazing fact is that when they returned to their normal weight, they spontaneously increased the amount of food to just the level necessary for them to sustain their weight. After all, overweight animals can't be found in their natural environment as the hunger and satiety mechanisms function just as nature intended: to maintain perfect harmony and balance. It is likewise with the human body: guiding it to choose food of high nutritional value through a proper nutrition plan will help the body restore its normal hunger and satiety mechanisms and this will be the first important step towards the ultimate achievement of normal weight."

1.4.2 Second Meeting: March 21, 2006

1.4.2.1 A relationship of trust

The 2nd meeting was crucial for her to build a relationship of trust with us. It was essential to create a feeling of trust. At this meeting, she negotiated confidence. We also explained the necessity for her to change the balance when trying to control her emotions, that is, to strengthen her emotional restraint. Failure to express what she feels triggers loss of control over food, which must be reversed. During the session she also talked about how protective she is towards her mother. Finally, she told us that after our first meeting, she left with a headache which she had also felt during that meeting. This is indicative of how much she internalises the tension.

Regarding the nutritional part, we noticed through her diary that she had begun taking control of her nutrition. She expressed that she felt much more revitalised, had got a better rest, that she woke up in a better mood and that now that she is better at organizing her meals and is rarely in a state of intense hunger. These recordings were extensively discussed, and essential observations were made on how next time, things could be better regarding the intake of more nutrients during the day and with slight changes she might reach mealtimes feeling less hungry. (At the end of Chapter 1, some features of the diaries kept throughout these 5 meetings are listed.)

1.4.3 Third Meeting: March 28, 2006

1.4.3.1 Desire for something better

The feeling that we had understood her difficulties brought her to the 3rd meeting, where she spoke more comfortably about her hardships. Our relationship of trust had started being established and the fact that she was able to trust anyone was particularly significant and comforting. It was also important that she was building a healing relationship within a protected environment. Within this relationship she could rely on someone and ask for help whenever she was afraid to act. She characteristically stated that she had never imagined she could have a binge-eating episode and feel no guilt, but mainly that she could report it to her dietitian without the fear of being reprimanded. She then stated that, through this new process, she was allowed to learn something different, take better care of herself and that for the first time she realized that food was not the means of dieting or decompressing her emotions. She also found it very comforting that we did not comment on her weight.

1.4.4 Fourth Meeting: April 4, 2006

1.4.4.1 Control and limits

In the 4th meeting we dealt with ways of controlling over-eating, because we had already noticed in the previews meeting that she was beginning to manage the episodes of over-eating that she had been having late at night. So, we wanted her control to become more organized and conscious. Having taken over, she had already began feeling more confident and hopeful that she would take matters into her own hands again. Some techniques that she had already implemented were:

a. choosing what went into her home, that is, not buying things that would entice her, so this was an essential preventive measure against relapse and new crises,
b. having decided that she wanted to take care of herself, so her motivation was clear.
c. hearing her inner voice that set a limit, which she had not previously listened to or even sabotaged. So, it was as if she had started cooperating with herself to be successful.

Also, she used the "voice of limitation" in other areas. She tried to set limits in her relationships with others and regarding what she did not want to do, either because they were pressing or emotionally charging for her. So, she began to realize that she should not tolerate everything, "she should not be able to do it at all," she did not need to be superhuman, and had to respect herself and her needs.

She also began to realize that under challenging times, eating is really a loophole. Through it, she avoided confronting her feelings or events in their actual foundation. But she did not want to live like that, so she decided that she did not want to avoid reality through eating.

What she learned from that day's meeting was that she was "aware of it", meaning she was aware of an upcoming binge eating episode. Anticipation gives her a chance to grow inside, a way out, while food is a quick and primitive reflex or respond to her fears but bringing no resolution to them.

An issue she got support for during the treatment is that we showed her that she is a human being who is eager to move forward and can quickly absorb and utilize new knowledge.

Her relationship with her mother was also discussed at this meeting. Their relationship with food largely explained her weight problem. Her mother was very greedy, and there was generally a culture of escaping through food in their household. On the other hand, her mother often blamed her for her body, saying, "Why do you look like this? Look at how much your belly has grown." This was a trap, a double bind that inhibited her. Through the treatment, we helped her see and deal with it by using expressions like, "Mother, on the one hand, you say I have a big belly and on the other you give me more to eat, what is my position in all this?"

An essential piece of information she gave us about her relationship with her mother is her mother's anxiety over her own mother's life. This should be treated with utmost respect, but at the same time, it introduces a great deal of confusion. The woman is burdened with anxiety for her mother and her mother, in turn, with that for her own mother. And the main focus here is to recognize it's right not to be able to manage everything. She must finally learn to admit that she cannot be perfect and do so without feeling guilty, which sets her back on her progress.

1.4.4.2 Last meeting's objectives

Before the last meeting, a little more time was given to for her to better understand what had taken place during the preceding ones and the meeting was scheduled a few days after Easter Sunday. The last session's purpose was to end with an evaluation of what she had gained through these meetings, new information she had received, what had helped her. She seemed in need to take care of herself even if she didn't do it by herself. We will also see what made it difficult for her to seek help, and where the difficulty lies, preventing her from taking care of herself now. It is also essential to recognize that one of her main obstacles is that she wants to please others.

We will focus on the fact that controlling her crises has raised her self- esteem, boosted her morale, given her hope, relief, and joy, and set her on a better path. We will empower what she has already achieved: regain control of the procedures that need to be followed until the new way of life has been fully adopted. All the despair that these people find themselves in results from the fact that they have lost control. This doesn't concern eating alone however, the same went for life generally. She was starting to control and improve situations that made her life difficult and to fortify her position and opinion.

1.4.5 Fifth Meeting: April 26, 2006

During the last meeting, we focused on prevention, in other words, how not to lose what had been achieved up to that point. We investigated how she had lost weight and how she had regained it in the past. We understood that when she lost weight, she would withdraw within herself, become isolated, and then gain weight again. She was essentially locked in a feeling, a situation, a single solution as if there was nothing else to think about, as if there was no alternative way to deal with occasional difficulties. One way to increase her weight was through anger and standing off against other people. If anyone told her: "You have to lose weight," she, on the rebound, would gain weight and vice versa. This behaviour was very frequent in her relationship with her mother, who kept telling her to lose weight. As the second child of the family, she had to stand up for her rights and claim them using her body, that is, by gaining or losing weight. What was suggested through therapy was working out a way to claim things without using her body to do so. But she had to understand that people pay attention to her because she has a respectable opinion and attitude, not because of her body size. For example, she was angry with men because they only look at physical appearance, still, this is the means she used to approach them; what she showed them; she did not let them see her inner world. This was a bitter truth and hearing it was not easy for her. She had been rejected too many times. This rejection made her double down, angry, and worsened the situation. What would help her was separating herself from her body as she could not seek a relationship by projecting the issue of weight or taking out her anger about it, that is, she had to clarify the relationship level in her mind.

Another essential issue was that when something negative happened in her life, no matter what she had done by then, she felt "empty." She forgot everything extraordinary she had previously achieved and felt like an insignificant person. At this point, we wanted to highlight her achievements. Specifically, we asked her to tell us the five most important things she had achieved in her life and felt proud of. Unfortunately, she said almost nothing either because she was uncomfortable or because she couldn't find anything to say at the time. What she mentioned as an achievement was that she was not afraid of life but what really seems to be happening to her was that she had no sincere contact with fear. She got terrified and when that happened, she put on weight. So, it was imperative to change, open up, find other ways of expressing herself apart from food, and find alternatives within herself.

It is important for her to always be vigilant and think that there are other things that come along with her successes, e.g., being happy, but also always be mindful and aware that there may be negative things behind any success. She should be frequently vigilant that there are still imponderables that she may not be able to control. When starting to lose weight again she should be careful not to be over-optimistic. It'd crucial for someone close to her to say, 'Did you manage it? Good! Keep the chances of recurrence in mind." Having a fear of being obese again would benefit her. It will help her protect herself. And when she reaches the point where she will have managed to do so, it is also possible that she will briefly go through anorexia until she finds her balance.

We also talked about establishing things that a "good" obese person does not do. The essence is to lose weight while developing new skills. She cannot lose weight without doing so, otherwise, it is only a matter of time before a relapse takes place. She has to build something new where old habits stood at the same time; otherwise, it will turn into another symptom (psychosomatic) e.g., she may lose weight and develop asthma or allergies, which this is very common occurrence.

Closing, we focused on developing alternative and complementary solutions. We consider exercise to be necessary, but we believed that exercising in a gym would not be suiting for her. Particularly for this woman, because stress was extremely intense in her daily life, yoga or Pilates would help her on multiple levels as she would be taught stress control techniques, and the dynamics of these exercises would help her body, worn out as it was by all previews diet attempts, improve in many levels.

Some simple methods of behavioural modification that could help people with an eating disorder maintain a well-balanced diet plan are daily light physical exercise, about thirty minutes a day, a relaxing massage session, reading an enjoyable book, using their imagination, relaxing music, a calming bath, socializing, praying, developing new hobbies and more.

We also believe that continuing to work with a psychotherapist would be a great help as there still were many issues that needed resolving and most importantly, strengthening her position as much as possible when it comes to people in her immediate environment (family, working, emotional) who clearly seemed to still have the power to negatively influence her.

Finally, with regard to her relationship with food, it would take a long time of cooperation with the psychologist and dietitian, no less than six months, until she would reach a sufficient level of ability to control her binge eating episodes. A part of the therapeutic expectation is having these episodes and at the same time, enjoying them. This results in not feeling guilty the next day but realizing that it is a new day, another opportunity for her to take care of herself.

After all, an important observation she made for herself is that even though she hadn't felt like she was on a diet in the weeks between meetings, she still felt her body improving, her clothes looser, her skin softer, her face having a more pinkish colour and, generally, her strength increasing. Thus, it was reaffirmed once again that the role of nutrition is vital in every positive change and in every new achievement we want to accomplish. It is clear that the methodology we applied through the prompt: "First eat all that can benefit you and then, whatever else your body or mind or senses want" can bring about any form of healing effort and expectation sooner. According to the ancient Greeks, the saying "A healthy mind can only dwell in a healthy body" has always been valid.

1.5 Treatment Methods and Techniques for People with Eating Disorders

1.5.1 Troubleshoot Issues Such as Minor Mistakes, Misconduct, Slips, and Derogations from the "Laps" Program

1.5.1.1 Regular meetings for the timely prevention of difficulties

During the last meeting, we provided enough information on possible relapse and its prevention. Several months after the end of the first five meetings, she still visited her dietitian, no longer on a weekly basis but every two or three weeks, because she had the information she needed and had already lost four kilos in the first two months without any special or stressful effort, just by taking advantage of what she already knew.

1.5.1.2 De-stigmatisation meetings

Suppose she comes to an appointment having had a relapse and knowing what went wrong, we should make sure that the relapse is de-stigmatised and has stopped there. It is essential for her to keep in touch even if she has grossly exceeded her diet plan. She should in no way abandon the meetings with her dietitian. At the same time, she should feel comfortable and admit, at any time, that something has gone wrong and that she has made a mistake. She should not hesitate, not blame herself anymore and try to talk about the reason why she has got out of track. For example, we knew that she exceeded the limit when she was isolated, so we had to prevent her from acting this way.

1.5.1.3 A reminder of the situations that sabotage the effort

It was important to remind her that she went out of line when she withdrew from people, her friends and her activities. She had to somehow stop, and we had to remind her again of what she had told us and recognized as inhibitive for her efforts.

1.5.2 Techniques for Dealing with Possible Deterioration, Interruption of Treatment, Return to an Earlier Worst State and Relapse

1.5.2.1 Reassess the new status

When she relapsed and hadn't shown up for some time, we had to reassess her situation. Since she was a person who took on other people's responsibilities, we had to see when she had started not taking care of herself. We needed to help her take a step back and realize that she has been burdened with other people's responsibilities and cares and should begin taking care of her own needs.

1.5.2.2 Reassessing stress

We also needed to reassess her stress levels or whether fatigue might have been affecting her. That is, to reassess the current situation and mainly look for any new conditions such as loneliness, boredom, frustration, romantic relationships, perhaps an additional personal frustration with a significant other and eating being a new self-punishment for failure, telling herself phrases like: "See? Things aren't working the way you are." To investigate if she is in another stage of life e.g., if she had got married, moved house, divorced, got pregnant, changed jobs, found herself unemployed, and generally in any stressful situations.

1.5.2.3 Have someone nearby taking care of her

When she "slipped" it was crucial to have a person, she felt close to, caring for her. That is, we had to check if there was someone to support and stand by her, who would urge her to go back to meeting her dietitian when they realised she wasn't able to make it, help her stick to the therapy, or get back into it as soon as possible, so that she wasn't left on her own to fight it. It was important for her that an expert should perform a deep investigation of the new situation and support her without causing guilt.

1.5.2.4 Relapse has always got something to say

Sometimes relapse has something new to say. An event that we probably haven't taken into account or didn't really pay much attention to in our last meeting. It is presented as a difficulty and points to something we must see. We need to use relapse to see what the new matter is that we didn't realize the previous time, that is to learn something from it so that it is not a mistake followed by guilt, but an opportunity for us to get new information. This requires feeling accepted, comfortable, and daring to attend the sessions even when they have made a mistake.

1.5.2.5 The constant reminding of the place where she had been taken care of in the past

An essential method that our experience has shown is helpful in bringing back people who for some reason have stopped a diet program is constantly reminding them of the place from which they once received help, e.g., by receiving greeting cards from us two to three times a year. For the Diatrofi science team, especially in recent years, the most frequent return of older customers has taken place since the bi-monthly distribution and posting of the journal Diatrofi. Health & Wellness began, the first thing people say being: "Every time I looked at the magazine outside my door, I felt that you still remember me and that I had to give myself another chance."

1.5.2.6 "Weight targeting" a vast topic for discussion

One of the most significant issues that an up-to-date dietitian has to address is the following complex situation: a client who, through appropriate diagnostic tests and experience, has been found to be suffering from some type of eating disorder and is asked to provide answers to the question of weight, set during the first session. The key questions the customer always asks are three: How much weight they will lose each week, the weight they need to reach, and finally, how long it will take to reach their desired weight. This is the time when the dietitian must unleash all his virtues, knowledge and patience to convince his client that being a person with an eating disorder, the last thing they should be thinking about is weight loss, for their health's sake.

1.5.2.7 Debunking a myth

Nowadays, modern nutrition science possesses effective means of evaluating total body weight. Through constants, we can explain the ideal percentages (but also their range) of not only fat but also muscle mass, bone mass, hydration, etc. Essential tools that have rid us of the antiquated "American Metropolitan Life Insurance Company" chart, where women had to be 10 pounds less than their second decimal height figure in meters, and men weighing close to their second decimal height figure in meters, e.g., a woman with a height of 1.65m should weigh up to 55 kg. A man with a stature of 1.80m should have a maximum weight of 80 kg. For the record, this chart was compiled after a statistical study revealed that when the clients of a certain insurance company had certain weight figures correlating to their stature, the company was less likely to pay the premium for possible medical care. This is an unacceptable chart that, unfortunately has been engraved so deeply into modern people's minds that it could only be removed by a lobotomy operation.

1.5.2.8 When the weighing scales gets stuck (weight loss "plateau")

As for the weighing scales "getting stuck", there are many ways for the dietitian to either interpret or deal with such cases, which is a huge topic for us to discuss. But we will try to provide an interpretation in simple and straightforward terms. Huge issues begin when the only way of controlling the progress of weight reduction is through weight monitoring using the weighing scales. It seems to get stuck or does so for long time periods, in the majority of cases with numerous weight fluctuations. But what never stops (as long as, there are no major unresolved hormonal problems) is the body's change for the better. Specifically, when a weight loss effort is combined with exercise and especially weightlifting or swimming.

Increasing muscle mass (usually reduced by previous unbalanced diets) and improving body hydration by eating more water-rich foods have the combined effect of positively increasing body weight by naturally enhancing the metabolic rate of the body. After all, as oil floats in water, so does human fat, it being the lightest part of the body. Fat has the largest volume and weighs less than all other parts of the human body.

For example, a dehydrated and unfit client who will follow our guidelines for proper nutrition and physical activity may have lost 2 kg of fat after one month, have gained 1 kg of muscle mass and rehydrated by 1 litre. The result is that the weighing scales show no difference in weight, but the client has already come down one size.

These measurements are evident if the dietitian uses techniques such as the "Body Independence Analyser" or even a skin fold calliper. That is why we consider it not merely important, but ESSENTIAL not to determine the progress of weight loss based on weighing scales but on the change of all body measurements. A simple measuring tape can provide great results, but also the constant reference to how the customer feels about his/her clothes in each visit i.e., if they feel more comfortable in them or if they buy smaller sizes than before, can be indicative of the excellent achieved result.

Another critical point is that the weighing scales getting stuck can also mean the need for a short pause to allow time for the psychological assimilation of the changes. People who have lost a lot of weight abruptly, due to the fact that this change did not happen at the same time with the change in body image, have often had the tragic effect of them regaining their original weight.

Some new theories claim that for every 5% reduction in initial weight, a pause of at least 15 days is necessary for the client to get familiarized with this body change. Also, the dietitian should often be ready to acknowledge and accept that the client may not be in the mood or may not have the strength to continue when they notice that their weight hasn't changed. Very often, a short break in the diet can be relieving but always in combination with healthy eating habits. In other words, we might consider this pre-agreed period as a "maintenance rehearsal." When there is constant pressure from themselves, their environment or the dietitian to continue the diet, the results are exactly the opposite, and the client relapses.

1.5.2.9 Ensuring environmental support

Unfortunately, most people with bulimia are women. A large percentage of them are women who are in a permanent relationship, such as marriage. The support from the partner or spouse is critical, so before commencing any form of treatment, their opinion should be heard, their position expressed as straightforwardly as possible, they mainly ought to be informed about the form of treatment, as well as the reasons why it is essential. In many cases, we may be able to convince a client suffering from an eating disorder that, at that stage, we should focus on improving their eating habits and not losing weight. On the other hand, the following paradox often appears: a partner or spouse who has not been adequately informed will insist that the reason their partner has gone to the dietitian is to lose weight and will understandably expect the coveted results every week. Proper and complete briefing to both couple members will help our joint effort with the client. We need to know if the partner or spouse will be supportive, whether they are worried or not, whether they will help and how they are thinking of helping; we will have to indicate ways how this is preferable to be done and which is their own responsibility in this joint effort. It is therefore vital, from the beginning of the treatment, that everyone be adequately informed about the importance of the condition and the course that is to be followed until the individual can get rid of the eating disorder and begin taking control of their eating. It is also important to ask for the partner's consent to be an ally in the treatment and they need to be informed on how much their partner needs their support to complete what they are starting. Usually, family members who are unaware of the difficulties of such a venture often sabotage the effort and make it difficult for both the client and the dietitian to work. It is imperative to clarify to all family members that everyone's diet needs to be adapted to that of the member who needs help. We should also consider the possibility that the husband or partner is not willing to be helpful or does not wish to work in the therapeutic framework we are building with our client. If this is the case, it is imperative to distinguish early on, whether the husband or partner can help her or the family in general. If they cannot, at least, the client must learn to recognize when and who can sabotage their effort so that they are always prepared and equipped with the skills to deal with it.

1.5.2.10 Other Psychological Parameters relative to Body Image

The point here has to do with how one relates his problems to his body, and essentially what is necessary is to reconstruct the idea that the body is a part of the whole and does not consist the whole. That is, the woman suffering from an eating disorder should begin to realize on the one hand that her body is not responsible for all the problems she faces and, on the other, that she should not take it out on her body when she faces problems and that she should stop treating it like a trash bin that swallows everything that happens. Of course, it takes a lot of work, both cognitive and emotional, for a person with an eating disorder to repair his or her image.

Evi's example is a typical case of a woman suffering from an eating disorder and is often an isolated person whose relationships with others are not easy. If she starts to see that all her problems are not owed to her weight but to the issues she faces within the context of having relationships with other people, maybe we can help her by giving her some perspective on how to function within relationships rather than isolating herself from them. That is, if she feels angry or disappointed in a relationship, we can point out that she doesn't help by being emotionally charged but by trying to work out a solution inside her, by working within the relationship, solving the problem there instead of taking it out on food. There is no need to swallow it, that is to start coming out of the isolation she is in, supressing her emotions by eating and start placing each matter in its rightful place. In this sense, it helps her to recognize that her body is not the only problem. To be successful, she also needs to acquire some new skills on relationships. She has to learn how to get into and to function in a relationship because it is common that a woman with an eating disorder does not know or has forgotten how to do this and wants actual help.

1.5.2.11 A healing relationship

I believe that several things have already been mentioned in the preceding pages about how dietitians should handle such situations. I hope that it is understood that in our relationship with the woman -or man- who suffers from an eating disorder, we should be patient and make them feel that we will be allies in this challenging effort. We also need to know they will test us, check if we can manage to stay in this relationship without being disappointed and most importantly, know that whatever they do she should not feel guilty and know that no one will blame them. It is also essential they keep in mind that we know that there will be setbacks in this race. Still, most importantly, with our help and support, they will manage to have more victories than defeats at the end. Knowing that if she ever loses control, her dietitian will always be by her side to help her and explain that even through a relapse, we will find an opportunity to learn something new to better future proof ourselves. I also consider very important and comforting, something that has to do with the original agreement a dietitian makes with his client regarding banned foods. It is preferable if our customer has a powerful desire for some food, to include it in the diet and relieve that desire rather than secretly reinforcing the vicious cycle of guilt so that even the most fattening foods can be seen as acceptable.

I find essential that all customers keep a daily record of the food they consume and under what conditions they consume it (place, with a company or alone, degree of hunger, emotional state, thoughts, level of physical activity) just like in the diary that will be described below.

1.5.2.12 A helpful relationship

Before going into a more detailed analysis of the nutrition policy against bulimia, I would like to give my opinion on the relationship between the two therapists for eating disorders, namely the dietitian and the psychologist. Studying all the above may have given the impression that dietitians should often substitute the psychologist, which I will try to further rectify in the next few pages. The boundaries of the dietitian and the psychologist must be very clear. No dietitian, no matter how good they may be, can handle any incident safely due to lack of proper training. But I do agree that they need to be sufficiently informed to understand their client's emotional state. On the other hand, and as it will be shown later, I find treating a person suffering from an eating disorder very difficult without the contribution of an adequately chosen dietary scheme.

I also believe that the dietitian can play an essential role in motivating the client to find many ways of getting rid of his or her problem and move towards a better and high-quality future. Since the dietitian develops a relationship and bonds with the client, if within that relationship the client does not feel that his or her dietitian understands or empathises with them or that they have a human connection, they will interrupt the therapy, burdening themselves with yet another failure, with the tragic consequence of additional psychological and thus physical weight. The more cultivated the dietitian is internally and spiritually, the more they will withstand, the greater the understanding they will show, thus the client will feel safe and trust them. That is why we need continuous education, cultivation and effort to constantly be up-to date. But I consider even more important the full experience a dietitian can gain by having a constant collaboration and communication with a psychologist to seek help and supervision for severe cases.

1.5.2.13 In the end, can anyone guarantee joy and happiness only through a successful outcome?

The most certain answer to this question is "this is a good question." It is a concern both of the client and the dietitian. The client wonders if the therapist can actually help him, hoping that they will not be another small paragraph in his long dietary resume. On the other hand, it is the therapist's, and especially the dietitian's, stress that really wants to help his client but always wonders if they will eventually be able to convince the patient that they are "the chosen one" who can achieve this, and even more importantly, if they will manage to follow him not only all the way until the end but to succeed in helping him maintain the target weigh after their common effort. This is definitely the biggest challenge.

From my own experience, I have come to realize that when a person with either an eating disorder or just a little extra weight, starts to change his or her eating habits, has found the communication he needs, and has begun to have a successful relationship, then he will start being happy, less scared of people, and feeling better and better. He will begin thinking that finally, having a meaningful relationship with the people around him is not the most challenging thing in the world. One last thing that may seem a bit metaphysical but often works, is to urge the client to envision his ultimate goal (his dream-goal), to remember past times when he was what he wants to become again. To think back through this process on how things were, the situations and the people around him when they were thinner, and to try with us to find ways in which they could bring back to the forefront and in his daily life some of the situations of the good old past. And why not do this ourselves: envision our client the way he imagines he will be happy and satisfied.

1.5.2.14 When is a person actually ready to start a diet?

Many people start a diet for the wrong reasons:

- For another person, such as their spouse, a boyfriend, their mother, etc.
- Negative body image (they hate their body instead of respecting it).
- For some special occasions, such as a holiday or a wedding, the decision is usually taken at the last minute, expecting

immediate and quick results, not taking into account the physical but also financial cost.

- They are determined to lose weight without realizing that they need to alter their behaviour, definitively changing their eating habits.
- They are convinced that losing weight will cure compulsive over-eating while in fact the abrupt deprivation of food will do just the opposite.

1.5.2.15 Is it the right time?

There are, of course, many reasons why people find it difficult to lose weight. Some of the factors that affect such an attempt are the person's body type, genes, the local society, and the individual's psychological condition. A key factor regarding psychology is someone's readiness to start a diet. Sometimes the circumstances are appropriate and other times they are not. The chances of success are greater if it is the right time for the person.

1.5.2.16 What does "being ready" mean?

Readiness refers to whether a person is ready to commit to a diet plan when starting to follow it. It relates to his mental state, motivations, and other factors that determine whether the time is right. People rarely wonder, "Am I ready to do this?"

Starting a diet when you are not really ready can be a problem, and you are likely to regain the lost weight. Losing weight and regaining it, also known as a "yo-yo" diet, can have health implications so people who regain weight may feel unsuccessful. They are ashamed when they are with people they know, feeling as if they need to apologize. Additionally, some are ashamed of having lost control.

Another critical issue is the impact that regaining weight has on subsequent weight loss efforts. It reduces people's confidence in whether they will ever succeed. After the joy of losing weight, regaining it can be psychologically devastating, striking a severe blow to morale.

1.5.2.17 Why is it important for someone to be ready?

Someone who wants to slim down is like someone who wants to climb to the top of a mountain like that of the "roof of the world." It's possible, but hard work is needed.

A smart person waits for the right circumstances. There is a difference between someone who sets off on a sunny weather and someone who does so in a thunderstorm. Climbers are well aware of the importance of proper weather conditions. However, many people who want to lose weight rush into the diet without thinking about whether their venture is likely to be successful.

This is one aspect of psychology, known as "denial". Self-pity is a feeling that usually drives people to a limited diet but, for at that time they refuse to think about the possibility of failure because they feel it will diminish their initial excitement.

Two aspects of readiness are essential:

- The first is to make people appreciate how important it is.
- The second is to assess an individual's readiness.

1.5.2.18 Discovering the real motives

How truly motivated the person is. Most people would reply, "Of course I'm motivated. I just need to lose some weight. I don't fit in my clothes. I can't bear to look at myself in the mirror ..." etc.

A good idea is to rate yourself from 1 to 10. Think of past efforts and rate yourself thinking of them. Is anything specific happening at this time? If not, can you do something to change this?

1.5.2.19 Commitment is half the battle

It refers to how long motivation will last, that is, the time required for adopting new eating habits. Losing some weight and not regaining it means that in the beginning, this process will last for some time and then the changes will be integrated in one's eating behaviour forever. Many people believe that weight loss is enough to keep this process going. Still, most of us dealing with obesity know that this is not true. And this becomes evident by numerous cases of people who regain the weight the have lost, soon after a treatment.

Commitment is the awareness that many of one's favourite habits should be limited. Habits they were likely to have held on a regular or daily basis should be set on a new foundation, such as limiting consumption of one's favourite sweets or high-calorie snacks and minding the choices one makes when going out to eat or going to a party, even the type and frequency of having fast food delivered. Can a person see himself or herself continue to do so in the span of three or six months?

Through discussing and training with the dietitian, thoughts and questions should be expressed like the following: "There are so many things that can affect the course of your diet, such as the attitude and behaviour of the people around you. There is always the possibility that they will not help you or sabotage your efforts."

There are many reasons people try to avert the efforts of those determined to follow a diet. Maybe they feel threatened or jealous when someone takes control of an aspect of their life or they may wish to have a person as a companion in their abuses, who going on a diet, will not be a part of the group anymore.

The last thought and consideration that to the potential client should be concerned with is: "Whatever the case, however things turn out, do you feel like you have the power to see yourself in control of situations like when someone says "help yourself, having one won't hurt" or "don't be boring" or "are you on a diet again?" will you be able to resist and cope?"

An excellent tactic to assist a dietitian who does not find the appropriate support (especially when the person is a young child or a teenager) comes with a question that the nutritionist poses in his or her environment:

"If there was an alcoholic person in the family, would there be drinks in the house?"

The automatic answer is "no".

"So why should a person who needs to restrain anything that may entice him to stray from his diet be constantly tempted? What I want from those of you around him today is to get everyone thinking that you have a person in the family who needs help, and that to really help them you will have to remove anything that would disrupt the schedule and his/her self-restraint. From now on you should avoid consuming takeaway food in the house, such as burgers, pizzas, etc. unless after consultation with his dietitian, these foods can occasionally be incorporated into his diet. To aid the member who is on a diet, it is important the whole family eat in the same way, and if another member wants to eat something different, to do so outside the house."

1.5.2.20 Under what conditions does the diet begin?

Our life often goes through different stages, sometimes less and sometimes more unpleasant or stressful. Starting a diet when one's life is in a transitionary stage can easily cause disruptions and make those around the person less tolerant.

Some characteristically disorganising situations are going through a divorce, relationship problems, an illness within the family, difficulties at work, or a period of stressful examinations such as exams to enter university. This, of course, does not always apply. For example, someone who leaves behind an unpleasant relationship may be highly motivated to lose weight and start a new life.

Someone starting a diet needs to think about what will happen in the months ahead and how the upcoming events will affect their chances of success. Next, let's look at a test suggested in the Master Practitioner in Eating Disorders and Obesity training by the National Centre for Eating Disorders in Great Britain.

1.5.3 Diet Readiness Test

1.5.3.1 Goals and behaviours

1. Compared to other times, how determined are you to lose weight this time? (0-10)
2. How confident are you that you will stay focused on your weight loss plan for as long as it takes to achieve the goal?
   (Sure enough = 0, less sure = 3, uncertain = 5)
3. Considering all the external factors in your life (work, family, relationship, etc.), to what extent can you try to follow a diet?
   (High = 0, Medium = 3, Low = 5)
4. Think honestly, how much weight do you have to lose and how fast do you hope to lose it. Calculating a loss of half to one kilo per week, how realistic are your expectations?
   (Fairly realistic = 0, not realistic = 5)
5. Do you fantasize about your favourite foods when dieting?
   (Continue = 5, sometimes = 3, not = 5)
6. Do you feel angry, deprived, or distressed when dieting?
   (Often = 5, sometimes = 3, never = 0)
   External factors
7. When the conversation comes to a food you like, or you read something about it, do you want to eat it, even when you're not hungry?
   (Yes = 5, No = 0)

8. How often do you eat because you're actually hungry?
   (Often = 3, never = 5, when needed = 0)
9. Do you have trouble controlling yourself and not eating when your favourite foods are in the house?
   (Yes = 5, No = 0)

1.5.3.2 Binge eating control

If the following situations happened during your diet, would you be more likely to eat more or less immediately after and for the rest of the day.
(Much less = 4, less = 3, slightly more = 2, more = 5)

10. Even though you have said you will not have lunch, a friend persuades you to go out to eat. Are you easily convinced?
    (Yes = 5, No = 0)
11. You break your diet by eating something forbidden.
    (Yes = 5, No = 0)
12. You have adhered to your diet and tested yourself with a treat.
    (Yes = 5, No = 0)

1.5.3.3 Compulsive binge eating

13. Apart from meals at celebrations or during a night out, have you ever consumed a large amount of food and felt that you ate too much without controlling yourself?
    (Yes = 5, No = 0)
14. How often have you eaten something you hadn't intended to eat and felt terrible afterward in the last month?
    (Often = 5, sometimes = 3, never = 0)
15. Have you ever used laxatives or vomited or worked out excessively to make up for it?
    (Yes = 5, No = 0)
16. How often did you do this last year?
    (Often = 5, Occasionally = 4, Never = 0)

1.5.3.4 Emotional eating

17. Do you eat more than you would like when you have negative emotions such as anxiety, depression, anger, or loneliness?
    (Often = 5, sometimes = 3, never = 0)

18. Do you have trouble controlling the amount of food you consume even when you have positive emotions, e.g., at festivals or at an outlet or party with food?
    (Often = 5, Occasionally = 3, No = 0)
19. Do you have trouble controlling the amount of food you consume after a fight or a hard day at work?
    (Often = 5, Occasionally = 3, Never = 0)

1.5.3.5 Fitness

20. How often do you workout?
    (Often = 0, little = 3, never = 5)
21. How confident are you that you exercise regularly?
    (Very = 0, Not at all = 5)
22. When you think about gymnastics, do you have a negative image in your mind?
    (No = 0, yes = 5)
23. How confident are you that you can incorporate exercising into your daily routine?
    (Sure = 0, Uncertain = 5)

1.5.3.6 Discussion

Performing this test and discussing the results with someone who wants to start a diet is useful. There is no readiness score. One can be highly motivated but very negative towards exercising - a discussion on the importance of exercise and an investigation of the reasons why one is negatively inclined towards it may be necessary. Sometimes a small discussion can prove invaluable at the beginning of a diet.

This test can be useful and make the person seriously consider if now is the right time to start a diet. If failure can be avoided, the chances of the person doing better in a future effort are increased. They will get stronger if they are aware of what they are really called to face. This test can help some people become motivated because it will prepare them for various issues and difficulties that may come up.

The test should be used to motivate and not show someone what is not suitable for them. It is useful because it will allow him to focus on what he can do. In general, people should preferably start when the chances of success are higher.

1.5.3.7 2 Months later ...

A few weeks after my first meetings with Evi, I asked her to write something like a letter that would record her experiences from this process. At first, she openly expressed that this would be very difficult for her, but when I explained that this process would be used to teach, inform and help other people in the future, she quickly changed her mind. She didn't do it right away, but after taking some time to think about it, she came to my office one day, holding the following letter in her hands. I thank her wholeheartedly for her courage, and I present you the letter word for word just as Evi compiled it to help all of you and all of us.

1.5.3.8 A few words about me, Evi...

I have studied journalism - but, as life is unpredictable, I followed a different path. I exercised this profession for two years in the Greek press, and then I was hired as a civil servant, which I have been working as for the last twenty-two years. The public sector may not be as interesting, but I have found my peace.

1.5.3.9 A look back at my past

I am the second child of a traditional, middle-class Greek family. I experienced a problematic adolescence in an overprotected and yet oppressive environment. All the "joys" of my youth, I lived in fear and guilt since they were all forbidden until I graduated from high school.

Over the years I also accumulated bitterness sadness and frustration, along with a fair amount of body weight after I learned to resort to eating.

After high school, my appearance began to seriously concern me. I made several desperate attempts at losing weight, but soon afterward I gained more than I had lost. The causes were purely psychological, owed to various events that took place in my life (family problems, relationship issues, etc.), which despite always having recognised, I never discussed. Also, it had never crossed my mind that I could seek the help of an expert.

Along the way, came very difficult times for my family. Health problems, both curable, and not. The pleasant and unpleasant events in my life alternated, but unfortunately, the latter were more frequent and long-lasting.

The most pleasant thing in my life during the past years was that I managed to have my own place, my shelter, which radically changed my life.

Of course, weaning is more difficult when done later in life, so I needed a four-month period to adjust to new life.

At first, my home was full of people, and I thought I was starting to expand my social circle, but I felt intense loneliness.

This, coupled with my family's severe health problems, that I was called upon to face led me to gain 66 pounds in one year.

For the last 5 years I have been closely supported by my dietitian, who has failed only in applying a zipper to my mouth. But when he found that I had gained this weight in a very short time, which by no means happened accidentally during the time I had stopped visiting him out of shame and guilt, he told me that he was unable to help me anymore and recommended that I consult a specialist...

Of course, I refused maybe because I didn't want to deal with reality and the problem in its real stature. Then I started a serious weight-loss effort again to convince my nutritionist not to abandon me. But the miracle again lasted only for four days, and shortly after, I had severe weight fluctuations and bulimic episodes.

Four months ago, my nutritionist, my only supporter all this time, suggested that I visit a psychologist who would collaborate with him to deal with my problem.

Surprisingly, I accepted because I was beginning to realise my deadlock. I now believed that it was my only salvation and the only solution to my problem.

The meetings the three of us had were not many but they were quite constructive.

The psychologist, at times with a warm and friendly way and at other times a strict manner, managed to elicit various "thorns" in my soul, which I had never imagined had contributed to the consumption of large and inappropriate quantities of food, but I never thought I would confide in someone I wasn't close to.

Merely three months after those meetings – of myself, my psychologist and dietitian - I began to manage my eating. I was not always successful, meaning that I do not always consume proper foods, e.g., fruit, which are not to my personal preference. Sometimes, but fortunately, not often, I think of food in difficult times, but I do not resort to it. I started practicing what I learned in our meetings, applying techniques, etc. I am slowly transitioning to maturity; sometimes I struggle and put great effort into it and other times avoiding uncontrolled and inappropriate eating comes effortlessly.

And this summer, unfortunately, I lived through challenging situations without any pleasant alternation. We faced difficult things, health problems in my family.

I my effort to recover from a routine gall operation, I started feeling good about and do things for myself. I was even in love with a colleague I met at the hospital.

Unfortunately, this story didn't end well. Shortly afterwards, more severe health problems in my family came up, which I was called to deal with alone, completely neglecting myself.

During my recovery, I, did not receive anyone else's care and assistance, as an "autonomous and self-sufficient" woman, and afterwards felt the need to complain about it. As my psychologist once advised me, everything is conquered with effort and demand.

Today, having achieved a small weight loss I am trying to heal the rest of my wounds, as I am not in a particularly good psychological state.

Loneliness, which sometimes is intense, as well as the lack of a partner are two major causes of my poor mental state.

Also, I still haven't managed to get over feeling guilty, neither can I avoid feeling remorseful every time I refuse to do things for others. I usually refuse initially but then feeling victimised, I submit.

Finally, I feel that I should continue visiting my psychologist, to discuss with her.

It is also noteworthy that I receive frequent and systematic criticism for my appearance, rejection, and racism from people which I am not able to deal with very well.

I certainly have a long way to go before I can overcome some things, but I'm willing to fight it this time, asking for more help by those I trust.

1.6 Overview

It is important for the dietitian to know all the reasons why his client has become overweight apart from long periods of over-eating. He must reveal the reasons that led to the over-consumption of food and work with them, sometimes on his own, and others with the help of a psychologist to rule out their reappearance. The incident described in Part I simply serves as the trigger for more thoughts, more discussions, more ideas, and solutions. The modern dietitian should no longer treat his client as someone with unnecessary body fat by providing a unique solution in the form of a hypocaloric diet based solely on food equivalents but should look beyond them using his insight. It is important to realise that he is facing a person who has been led to obesity mainly by lack of emotional nutrition. This is the most significant gap his client needs to fill first. From this point of view, the position of the dietitian is particularly challenging as through the educational programs of the departments of food science and nutrition, he has not been trained for this purpose. On the other hand, he is the first recipient of this whole wave of futility pessimism and analgesia.

On the other hand, overweight clients should no longer treat dietitians as people who try to get them slimmer but as health scientists aiming to change and improve their eating habits.

Fighting eating disorders is clearly not an easy task for dietitians, which requires extra knowledge we would generally call "extracurricular" - beyond the curriculum of the food science and nutrition departments of the corresponding university schools. Obviously, a dietitian could never replace the professional experience and training of a psychologist or psychotherapist, but I think he can understand when his client's over-eating problem is triggered by factors other than excessive calorie intake or long-term unorthodox eating habits. The dietitian needs to master and utilise the results of specific diagnostic tests to identify at least the fundamental psychological aspects of his client that strengthen his eating disorder and difficulty with eating control.

Throughout my professional experience, I have often sought the help of a psychologist to understand the conditions under which the person standing in front of me was led to binge eating. Through meetings, such as those in Evi's case as well as many other similar cases, I have become able to better understand the people who sought my help seeking a better quality of life and with the psychologist's help and supervision, discovered new techniques of approach. But even then, when I asked some clients if they should seek help from a psychologist, I often encountered resistance as being treated by a psychologist is still a strong taboo in Greece. Many times, the solution to the opposition has been through a simple phrase: "the psychologist will help me help you." This phrase also was the key to the venture in Evi's case. The five meetings that took place in the psychologist's presence and the dialogues and conclusions that came up, answered essential questions and provided me with meaningful solutions to proceed with Evi and help her further. These meetings did not have a psychotherapeutic aspect for Evi, they were only meant to raise her awareness on the issues that had to do with everything causing her eating disorders. Throughout the meetings, we were able to focus primarily on a cognitive level, so that during every life stage she will be able to understand that each time she is led to a binge eating episode, it is actually caused by her need to fill an emotional vacuum. A large void that, due to lack of care or inability to be expressed when it was necessary, was buried under large quantities of food when the time was due. A typical phrase that perfectly illustrates this situation is "when I swallow my emotions... I eat something to help them go down".

It does not matter if, in any corresponding case, our client chooses before, after or during our cooperation to solve other issues that concern him and hold him back like an anchor impeding his personal progress towards a better quality of life. He may never get into this process. But at least he will have two things in his mind. Firstly, that he will have learned to distinguish when he eats due to hunger and when he does so to fill various emotional voids and secondly, he will always hold the knowledge that if at any time he wishes to come out of the various existential dreadlocks that deplete his opportunities for a happier life, there will always be an available opportunity. He will have the information that when he is alone with himself in front of his personal mirror, he will at some point finally have to work with himself seeking the help and assistance of the appropriate psychotherapist. After all, my personal opinion, and that of any health therapist, is that we all more or less need healing for our souls.

The following food diaries are indicative of Evi's dietary changes from the first, until the last days of our sessions. Their hourly recording during the day, simultaneously including the level of hunger and the correlating emotions that went along with it, undoubtedly reveal whether insufficient food intake can affect a binge-eating episode.

These diaries present deficiencies and deviations from the dietitian's model, presented in detail in Chapter 4.

Date: Sat 24/3/2007

Time	**Solid and liquid food**	**Degree of hunger (0-5)**	**Place and company**	**Emotions - thoughts**	**Important events**
9:00	1 cup of milk with 4 tablespoons of cereal with fruit, coffee	2	Alone at home		
13:00	1 fruit	2	Alone at home		
15:00	Pasta with tuna and salad	4	Alone at home		What different I expect from myself tomorrow
18:30	2 Flatbreads	4	Alone at home	Uncontrollable desire for food	
20:30	Hot chocolate	-	With a friend at a cafe	Intense dysphoria and weight from eating	
23:30	2 small pieces of dark chocolate				

Date: 25/3/2007					
Time	**Solid and liquid food**	**Degree of hunger (0-5)**	**Place and company**	**Emotions – thoughts**	**Important events**
10:00	1 cup of milk with 4 tablespoons of cereal		Alone at home		
13:30	Baked vegetables and potatoes and 2 small rusks. Coffee with a little milk		Alone at home while I was cooking.		
18:30	4 small pieces of spinach pie		Alone at home	Gluttony	What different I expect from myself tomorrow
22:00	A cup of green tea, a fruit				

Date: 26/3/2007					
Time	**Solid and liquid food**	**Degree of hunger (0-5)**	**Place and company**	**Emotions – thoughts**	**Important events**
6:30	A cup of milk, 3 small rusks		Alone at home		
11:00	Juice		At the office with colleagues		

12:30	A few salty almonds at a celebration (2 handfuls)		At the office with colleagues	Pleased because I resisted eating sweets.	What different I expect from myself tomorrow
16:00	Spinach with rice, graviera (a portion), 2 small rusks		Alone at home		
19:00	A resin bread		Alone at home		
21:00	A tangerine		Alone at home		
22:30	A piece of "bugatsa" (sweet cream in filo pastry)		Alone at home	Pleasure - My favourite sweet	

Date: 27/3/2007					
Time	**Solid and liquid food**	**Degree of hunger (0-5)**	**Place and company**	**Emotions - thoughts**	**Important events**
9:30	A cup of milk, 1 tablespoon of cereal, 2 rusks	2	Alone at home		
12:30	Meal. 3 small pieces of spinach pie	5	Alone at home		What different I expect from myself tomorrow
19:00	A small piece of "bugatsa"	2	At home with friends	Pleasant mood, as I am in good company	
21:30	A small piece of "bugatsa", a piece of spinach pie	3	Alone at home		

Date: 28/3/2008					
Time	**Solid and liquid food**	**Degree of hunger (0-5)**	**Place and company**	**Emotions - thoughts**	**Important events**
7:30	A sandwich	3	At the office alone		
13:00	Juice	4(thirst)	At the office with colleagues		
16:00	Pasta with tuna. 2 slices of bread	3	Alone at home		
21:30	Yoghurt with walnuts, fruit	2	Alone at home but coming back from a beauty salon.	Pleased for disciplining, while I was thinking of many "sinful" foods, I didn't give in	What different I expect from myself tomorrow

Date: 29/3/2007					
Time	**Solid and liquid food**	**Degree of hunger (0-5)**	**Place and company**	**Emotions - thoughts**	**Important events**
6:30	Yoghurt with walnuts, fruit 1 tablespoon of cereal	2	At home		
12:00	Juice	3	At the office		What different I expect from myself tomorrow
16:00	Pasta with tuna, bread	4	At home		

19:30	10 almonds, a juice	2	At home		
22:00	A little pasta with grated cheese, 1 rusk	3	At home	Emotionally charged after visiting my parents	

Date: 30/3/2007

Time	Solid and liquid food	Degree of hunger (0-5)	Place and company	Emotions - thoughts	Important events
8:30	As on 29/3				
12:00	A small sweet				What different I expect from myself tomorrow
13:30	juice				

Date: 31/3/2007

Time	Solid and liquid food	Degree of hunger (0-5)	Place and company	Emotions - thoughts	Important events
10:30	2 slices of cheese, 1 slice of ham, 2 rusks.	3	Alone at home		
12:30	Juice	2	Alone at home		
17:30	As in breakfast	5	Alone at home		

20:00	2 cups of green tea	-	With friends	In a good mood, talking about common issues.	What different I expect from myself tomorrow
21:30	Take out (Chinese, medium serving, variety)	3	With friends	As above. Actual hunger but didn't eat much.	

Date: 1/4/2007					
Time	**Solid and liquid food**	**Degree of hunger (0-5)**	**Place and company**	**Emotions - thoughts**	**Important events**
8:30	A cup of milk, 4 tablespoons of cereal with fruit, a small piece of tahini pie			I felt incomprehensible unrest and stress throughout the day. Finally, there were 2 occurrences that made me feel disheartened, under different circumstances I would have eaten uncontrollably, but I controlled myself. A phone call to a friend helped immensely, I got it off my chest.	What different I expect from myself tomorrow
12:30	Juice				
15:30	Roasted chicken with potatoes, salad				
20:00	A little Chinese takeout (a small plate)				

Date: 2/4/2007 (Monday before Easter)					
Time	**Solid and liquid food**	**Degree of hunger (0-5)**	**Place and company**	**Emotions - thoughts**	**Important events**
6:30	A cup of milk, 4 tablespoons of cereal and fruit.		At home		
12:00	Juice		At the office		
14:00	Tuna salad with boiled potato, boiled green beans, onion, parsley, 3 small rusks.		At home		What different I expect from myself tomorrow
20:00	A cup of green tea, almonds (medium quantity)		At home, in good company		
3:00	A banana				

Date: 3/4/2007 (Tuesday before Easter)					
Time	**Solid and liquid food**	**Degree of hunger (0-5)**	**Place and company**	**Emotions - thoughts**	**Important events**
6:30	A banana, 5 almonds	3	Alone at home	Stress about leaving for work in time.	Our meeting was constructive.
8:30	Half a piece of raisin cake	2	At the office with colleagues		What different I expect from myself tomorrow
12:30	Juice	2	At the office with colleagues		

15:30	Tuna salad and greens, 2 small rusks.	4	Alone at home	Pleased about resisting temptations.	To apply all I have learned in our meetings, techniques, etc.
21:00	A vegetable sandwich.	3	Alone at home	Pleased about resisting temptations.	

Date: 4/4/2007 (Wednesday before Easter)

Time	Solid and liquid food	Degree of hunger (0-5)	Place and company	Emotions - thoughts	Important events
6:30	A banana	3	Alone at home		
8:30	Half a piece of raisin cake	2	At home with colleagues	Good psychological mood, this is why I stopped at half the quantity of cake.	
11:00	A small mushroom pastry	-	At the office with colleagues	Small craving. I ate them consciously, I stopped at two pieces.	What different I expect from myself tomorrow
12:00	A small potato pastry	-	At the office with colleagues	As above	
15:30	A raw vegetable salad, 3 small rusks.	3	Alone at home	Resisted many "sinful" foods.	
20:30	A flatbread with 1 tomato.	3	Alone at home	Again discipline	

Date: 5/4/2007 (Thursday before Easter)					
Time	**Solid and liquid food**	**Degree of hunger (0-5)**	**Place and company**	**Emotions - thoughts**	**Important events**
9:30	A banana, a raisin bread			During the day I had some unpleasant thoughts, but I managed.	
14:00	Juice				What different I expect from myself tomorrow
15:00	Bean soup, salad, a slice of bread, 5 olives				
18:30	1 fruit				
21:00	1 fruit				
22:00	“Dakos” salad with mustard				

Date: 6/4/2007 (Friday before Easter)					
Time	**Solid and liquid food**	**Degree of hunger (0-5)**	**Place and company**	**Emotions - thoughts**	**Important events**
9:00	A cup of coffee, 2 rusks, a banana				
15:00	Raw salad				What different I expect from myself tomorrow

18:30	1 fruit				
23:00	Some nuts, 3 tablespoons of cereal				

Date: 7/4/2007 (Saturday before Easter)					
Time	**Solid and liquid food**	**Degree of hunger (0-5)**	**Place and company**	**Emotions - thoughts**	**Important events**
9:30	1 coffee, a cookie.	2	At my parents' house	Relief after holy communion	
12:00	1 fruit	4	At home	I feel pressed by all the unfortunate events in my life.	What different I expect from myself tomorrow
16:00	A raw salad with tuna, 3 rusks	4	At home		
00:30	2 pieces of cheese pie, salad, 2 eggs, 2 bites of potato, 1 rusk	4	In a family gathering.	Realisation that I cannot recognise, accept and enjoy the good things in life.	

Date: 8/4/2007 (Easter Sunday)					
Time	**Solid and liquid food**	**Degree of hunger (0-5)**	**Place and company**	**Emotions - thoughts**	**Important events**
10:00	A cup of milk, 4 tablespoons of cereal.				

14:00	1 portion of grilled goat with potatoes, 1 boiled egg, salad Flatbread with 1 egg, grated cheese, 1 tomato				What different I expect from myself tomorrow

Date: 9/4/2007

Time	Solid and liquid food	Degree of hunger (0-5)	Place and company	Emotions - thoughts	Important events
9:00	1 cup of milk, 4 tablespoons of cereal.		With friends	I have started feeling better, but I am still holding back.	
12:00	A bun.		With friends		
15:30	A little grilled meat, lamb chops, 1 small piece of bread, 1 large tablespoon of "Tzatziki", salad. A small piece of chocolate.		With friends		What different I expect from myself tomorrow
17:00	Natural juice		With friends		
18:30	10 almonds, green tea.		With friends		
20:30			Alone at home	Calm and relaxed.	

Date: 10/4/2007					
Time	**Solid and liquid food**	**Degree of hunger (0-5)**	**Place and company**	**Emotions - thoughts**	**Important events**
8:30	Half a serving of yoghurt, half a banana, 4 almonds, 1 tablespoon of cereal.	3	At the office with colleagues.	Joy and sadness.	
9:30	1 small chocolate tart.		At the office with colleagues.		What different I expect from myself tomorrow
12:30	A little juice		At the office with colleagues.	The more I work, the better I feel.	
14:30	1 grilled fish, salad, 1 slice of bread.	2	At my parents' home	Mixed feelings.	

1.7 Key Takeaways

1. **Understanding eating disorders is essential:** Disorders like bulimia and binge eating are not just habits; they are complex issues that require a holistic approach.
2. **The link between emotions and food:** Emotions often drive our eating habits. Feeling anxious or sad might lead to overeating or restrictive eating.
3. **The power of a food diary:** By tracking what you eat and how you feel, you can identify patterns that help you understand your relationship with food.

4. **Balancing hunger and fullness:** Your body's natural balance can be restored through nutrient-rich meals and healthy eating habits.
5. **Small changes make a big difference:** Focus on gradual behaviour changes. For example, add variety to your meals and choose foods with high nutritional value.
6. **Addressing societal and personal biases:** Embrace your body as it is and free yourself from stereotypes and negative beliefs.
7. **Stories for inspiration:** See how a holistic approach can bring real transformation through the eyes of other individuals who have had similar experiences.
8. **Strategies for empowerment:** Instead of letting negative emotions guide you, use them to develop positive actions and boost your confidence.

Chapter 2

The Nutritional Aspect of Treating Eating Disorders

Problems often work just like being in love...they go away leaving a gut as the aftermath.

2.1 Factors Influencing Hunger and Satiety*

2.1.1 When the Body Is Full, but the Mind Is Still Hungry

Hunger and satiety are fundamental aspects of human physiology, as well as for most living creatures. These mechanisms help organisms regulate their food intake to maintain a healthy balance in terms of nutrient intake and energy expenditure. In the animal kingdom, these mechanisms typically work flawlessly, preventing the occurrence of obesity. However, when it comes to humans, it seems like these mechanisms sometimes go awry, leading to deviations from the norm. In this exploration, we will delve into the intricacies of hunger and satiety, with a particular focus on two vital mechanisms: Serotonin and Glucose. This journey into the human body will reveal the miracles that occur within us, transforming the way we perceive food.

*Sections 2.1 and 2.2 are from the notes of *Professional Training Courses in Eating Disorders, Obesity & Nutrition* from NCFED, by nutritionist Mrs. Jane Nodder PhD.

Nutritional Intelligence: The Answer to Bulimia, Overeating, and Obesity
Evangelos Zoumbaneas

ISBN 978-981-5129-74-8 (Hardcover), 978-981-5129-73-1 (Paperback), 978-1-003-65188-8 (eBook)
www.jennystanford.com

Under normal conditions, humans possess a remarkable ability to automatically control and regulate the intake of various nutrients essential for their body. When the levels of these nutrients drop below a specific threshold, the body triggers mechanisms to restore the balance. This mechanism operates similarly to most animals, helping to maintain stable body weight. Even when presented with ample food, these creatures consume precisely what they need to sustain their weight. However, when it comes to conditions like bulimia, this delicate balance is disrupted, leading to uncontrollable food consumption. Bulimia represents an extreme deviation from the homeostasis that characterizes a balanced state, with unstable nutrient levels wreaking havoc on an individual's ability to control food intake. The ultimate goal of treating bulimia is to restore the balance between nutrient absorption and the body's natural chemicals, allowing the person to regain the ability to say "enough."

2.1.2 Dietary Deficiencies and Malnutrition

People following weight-loss programs or restrictive diets often experience the adverse effects of malnutrition. Low-calorie diets can resemble periods of voluntary starvation, creating confusion for the body. It struggles to differentiate between dieting and starvation, leading to adverse consequences. Prolonged dieting with repeated calorie restriction can result in severe health complications, affecting energy levels, mood, and weight. Inadequate nutrition causes physical disorder and biochemical imbalances.

According to the World Health Organization (WHO), malnutrition that approaches starvation occurs when daily calorie intake drops below 1200 calories. Despite this guideline, many individuals fail to consume sufficient food to meet their energy requirements, leading to paradoxical weight gain. The quality of calories consumed plays a crucial role, with sugar, white flour, processed foods, and saturated fats contributing to weight gain, despite their minimal nutritional value. Overeating nutrient-rich foods can also be problematic when the body cannot metabolize the excess.

The Impact of Skipping Meals and Calorie Restriction: Skipping meals or calorie restriction can lead to a range of issues. It disrupts blood glucose levels, resulting in low energy levels and stress. Chronic skipping of breakfast can even lead to the development of conditions like diabetes mellitus and mineral deficiencies. Deprivation of food and calories can also impact the thyroid gland's function, as the body attempts to protect itself from future periods of malnutrition by reducing metabolic rates. This can make subsequent weight loss attempts more challenging.

Essential Nutrients and Their Role: Essential fatty acids are crucial for brain function, hormone production, and stress management. Many individuals avoid dietary fats under the false belief that all fats contribute to weight gain. However, it is vital to prioritize sources of essential fats like olive oil, fish, and raw nuts in a daily diet.

Protein, another essential nutrient, plays a significant role in repairing damaged tissues and maintaining mental health. Inadequate protein intake can lead to mood changes, such as depression, anxiety, irritability, compulsive behavior, and low self-esteem. Additionally, when the body lacks carbohydrates, it resorts to consuming muscle tissue for energy, leading to a decrease in the basic metabolic rate and increased fat storage.

Pre-packaged Dietary Foods and Artificial Sweeteners: Pre-packaged dietary foods are often lacking in calories and nutrients, highly processed, and chemically loaded. They fail to provide the necessary nutrition the body requires.

Caffeine, when consumed in excess, can lead to symptoms of fatigue, nervousness, anxiety, and depression. It inhibits the production of serotonin and melatonin, impacting the body's ability to control food intake. Artificial sweeteners may contribute to the development of compulsive eating behaviors, as they can act as stimulants and interfere with serotonin production. Their consumption has been associated with a range of negative symptoms, including weight gain, headaches, depression, and anxiety attacks.

Low-Quality Vegetarian and Monophagic Diets: Low-quality vegetarian diets and monophagic diets, such as extreme detox programs, often lack essential nutrients, especially protein and vital minerals like iron and zinc. These diets can have negative effects on the thyroid gland and mental health. Vegetarianism is more common among individuals with eating disorders, which can be a symptom of the disease's psychopathology. Strictly vegetarian diets can pose unexpected risks, so incorporating dairy products is essential.

2.1.3 Conclusion

Hunger and satiety mechanisms play a crucial role in regulating food intake and maintaining a healthy balance of nutrients and energy in the human body. Deviations from these mechanisms can lead to various health issues, including malnutrition, weight gain, and mental health problems. Understanding the importance of balanced nutrition and the role of essential nutrients is essential for overall well-being. By recognizing the factors that affect hunger and satiety, individuals can make informed dietary choices to support their health and maintain a harmonious relationship between their bodies and the food they consume.

2.1.4 Prolonged Diet and Associated Risk Factors

Prolonged adherence to strict dieting regimens can lead to a range of adverse health effects and increase the risk of various conditions:

Gallstones: A strict diet with deficient daily calorie intake can result in an increased risk of gallstone formation. Approximately 25% of individuals on lean diets develop gallstones.

Diabetes Mellitus: There is an elevated risk of developing diabetes mellitus associated with prolonged dieting.

Reduced Sexual Desire: A decrease in sexual desire may occur due to nutritional deficiencies resulting from extreme dieting.

Mental Impairment: Mental functions can be impaired as a consequence of prolonged dieting, affecting cognitive abilities and overall mental well-being.

Risk of Cardiovascular Events: Prolonged dieting, especially when coupled with the use of diet pills, can heighten the risk of sudden heart attacks or strokes.

Reduced Life Expectancy: Overall, engaging in long-term, restrictive dieting practices may lead to a reduction in life expectancy.

2.1.5 Link between Nutritional Deficiencies and Eating Disorders

While not all individuals who skip meals or follow low-calorie diets will develop eating disorders like anorexia or bulimia, a connection exists between nutritional deficiencies and the risk of these conditions. Research published in the "British Medical Journal" revealed that adolescents following a strictly hypocaloric diet were eight times more likely to develop an eating disorder compared to adults on similar diets. This highlights the potential risks associated with extreme dieting.

Malnutrition stemming from a strict diet, as seen in anorexia nervosa, triggers a powerful response in the brain akin to the effects of opioids. Endorphins and other natural chemicals are released, providing a sense of pleasure, energy, and stress relief. In some cases, stricter diets intensify the desire for such restrictions.

Similarly, binge eating and vomiting, common behaviors in bulimia, can stimulate the release of endorphins, creating a mental dependency and an overwhelming urge to eat that is challenging to manage.

2.1.6 Nutritional Deficiencies and Thiamine

Thiamine, an essential B vitamin, cannot be synthesized by the human body and must be obtained through dietary sources such as pulses, whole grains, various grains, sesame, tahini, meat, and vegetables. Individuals with eating disorders, particularly anorexia nervosa, often develop thiamine deficiency. Early thiamine deficiency symptoms closely resemble those observed in the initial stages of anorexia nervosa. In cases of eating disorders like bulimia, where unorthodox diets and nutritional depletion are common, the risk of transitioning to anorexia increases, further jeopardizing physical and mental health. Thiamine deficiency can have profound consequences, emphasizing the critical role of nutrition in the development and progression of eating disorders.

2.1.7 The Role of Zinc in Eating Disorders

In the realm of nutrition, the importance of adequate zinc levels cannot be understated. Zinc deficiency shares some striking similarities with the symptoms observed in anorexia nervosa. This connection has prompted researchers and clinicians to consider incorporating zinc administration as part of the therapeutic approach. Achieving optimal zinc levels through food can be challenging, not only for individuals with anorexia nervosa but also for those consuming regular amounts of food. Zinc inadequacy is a prevalent concern.

Zinc-rich foods include red meat, egg yolk, whole grains, nuts, sunflower seeds, sesame seeds, and tahini. Nevertheless, despite these dietary sources, the exact role of zinc in treating eating disorders remains somewhat enigmatic. Research in this area is limited, with inconclusive findings. It is evident that eating disorders such as bulimia and anorexia are multifaceted, extending beyond zinc deficiency or adequacy.

In 2006, a novel mechanism was proposed to elucidate zinc's influence on neurotransmitters. A study by Birmingham and Gritzner in 1994 laid the groundwork for this hypothesis. It recommended a daily oral zinc supplement of at least 2 mg for all patients with anorexia nervosa. This suggestion aimed to address appetite disorders, mitigate binge-eating episodes in patients with binge eating and bulimia, alleviate depression, enhance energy levels, bolster physical and mental endurance, and restore healthy appetite and taste function. However, it is worth noting that the "National Institute for Clinical Excellence" (NICE Guideline 2004) in the United Kingdom does not advocate zinc supplementation as the sole dietary intervention during treatment.

2.1.8 Appetite Disorders and Brain Neurotransmitters

The intricate interplay of brain chemicals, known as neurotransmitters, shapes the neural networks governing our thoughts, emotions, and behaviors. These compounds exert a profound influence on how we perceive and respond to the world. An intriguing connection exists between the foods we consume and the levels of specific brain neurotransmitters. Notably, these brain chemicals can be several hundred times more potent than highly addictive substances like heroin and cocaine.

The chemistry that unfolds in the brain during binge-eating episodes closely mirrors the effects of simultaneously consuming alcohol and drugs. As individuals indulge in large quantities of food, particularly refined carbohydrates like sweets and starchy products, these "addictive foods" create a deceptive sense of fullness in the brain, cultivating dependency.

Crucially, several neurotransmitters significantly impact appetite and mood. Key players in this complex arena include catecholamines (e.g., dopamine, adrenaline, and noradrenaline), endorphins, and serotonin, each with distinct effects.

2.1.9 Prolonged Stress and Its Effects

Prolonged stress can deplete the brain's natural sedatives, tonics, and pain relievers, wearing down individuals who may already possess low levels of these protective chemicals due to genetic predisposition. The brain eventually struggles to cope with persistent demands, leading people to turn to food that relieves stress and elicits an addictive response.

2.1.10 Regular Consumption of Addictive Foods and Substances

Regular consumption of addictive foods, such as refined carbohydrates, or the use of substances like alcohol and drugs, has a profound impact on the brain's natural chemicals. Exogenous substances like alcohol and drugs attach to receptors meant for neurotransmitters, inhibiting and suspending the brain's natural chemicals. Over time, this can lead to a phenomenon known as "downregulation," wherein cells decrease the number of receptors to minimize sensitivity to a particular molecule. The brain becomes less responsive to its natural production of neurotransmitters, resulting in increased dependence on the external substance.

In essence, individuals replace their body's natural stimulants and relaxation agents with external substances, leading to the cessation of their natural production. Dependency on the substance gradually intensifies, mirroring the trajectory seen with drug use. Initially, a small amount is sufficient to achieve the desired effect, but over time, increasing amounts are required. Eventually, the substance takes control, and the user becomes subservient to it.

2.1.11 Impact of Light Exposure on Serotonin and Melatonin

The exposure to light plays a pivotal role in the synthesis of serotonin and melatonin in the pineal gland. Serotonin is converted into melatonin when darkness signals the need for sleep. Bright light, on the other hand, interrupts this process. Serotonin's smooth conversion to melatonin is essential for quality sleep. Inadequate serotonin production during the day can result in poor sleep quality, leading to persistent drowsiness and increased appetite.

2.1.12 Influence of Physical Activity on Neurotransmitters

Regular physical activity is a powerful ally in maintaining a healthy balance of neurotransmitters. Exercise requires energy, relieves stress, enhances mood, boosts self-esteem, and helps control food and alcohol cravings. Moderate exercise is especially beneficial in suppressing appetite.

Exercise can also stimulate serotonin production in the short term. During exercise, amino acids are directed toward muscle repair, while tryptophan, a precursor to serotonin, is readily introduced into the brain without competition from other amino acids used for muscle repair. Additionally, exercise increases oxygen uptake, a critical component in serotonin production.

In conclusion, understanding the intricate connections between nutrition, brain chemistry, and behavior is vital in comprehending the complex nature of appetite disorders. The interplay of neurotransmitters, genetic predisposition, stress, dietary choices, and physical activity all contribute to the multifaceted landscape of these disorders. Acknowledging the critical role of zinc and other factors can pave the way for a more comprehensive approach to managing and treating these complex conditions.

2.1.13 Regulation and Balancing of Brain Chemistry

The brain operates as a meticulous chemist, perpetually striving to maintain a harmonious balance of neurotransmitters. This intricate process ensures that the ebb and flow of these vital chemical messengers remains uninterrupted and that they are consistently available for use. The exchange of neurotransmitters between neurons is a constant requirement, and the brain regulates their quantities diligently. It deciphers messages sent through these fluctuating chemicals in its ceaseless effort to maintain the delicate chemistry of the mind. In essence, the brain is continually engaged in a balancing act. For individuals struggling with bulimia, this equilibrium proves elusive, making them imbalanced beings. Recognizing this fundamental truth is pivotal for both therapists and those afflicted by bulimia, as it paves the path to healing. The ultimate goal is the swift restoration of balance.

When the key neurotransmitters are present in adequate amounts, our mood and emotional state remain stable. Any disruptions in their balance can lead to either an insatiable desire for excessive food intake, primarily sweet or starchy foods, or a voluntary refusal to eat, which can override the physiological need for food. This can result in dependence on certain foods to trigger euphoria and restore a good mood.

2.1.14 Sugars and Amino Acids Nourishing the Brain

The brain's energy requirements are met by two unique fuels:

- Glucose: Derived from carbohydrate-rich foods, it significantly impacts blood sugar levels.
- L-glutamine: Naturally present in protein-rich foods, it is the most abundant amino acid in the human body. L-glutamine can swiftly supply the brain, often immediately curbing strong cravings for sweets and starches. This amino acid also stabilizes mental function, promoting calmness, alertness, and good digestion.

2.1.15 The Brain's Influence on Digestion

The presence of neurotransmitters in the digestive system, along with specific receptors, establishes the gut as an extension of the brain for certain purposes. This "intestinal perception" implies that the gut can have a say in our overall well-being. A well-functioning digestive system often plays a pivotal role in maintaining our mood. Incomplete food digestion, as seen in conditions like colitis or intolerance to specific foods, can send erroneous messages about hunger and satiety. Factors such as frequent antibiotic use and stress also impair the digestive system's proper function. A probiotic supplement, recommended by an appropriate therapist, can significantly improve both digestion and mood in individuals with indigestion.

2.1.16 Neurotransmitters and Appetite Control

Appetite control is governed by a multitude of neurotransmitters, each with its unique role. Some, like endorphins, noradrenaline, and neuropeptide Y, increase appetite, while others, such as cholecystokinin, serotonin, and corticotrophin, help reduce the desire for food.

Cholecystokinin (CCK): Cholecystokinin is one of the neurotransmitters that reduce appetite. It is elevated as food travels to the duodenum, leading to a progressive sense of fullness after a meal. A simple tactic to enhance CCK levels and quell appetite is to stand up during a meal, such as walking for a minute after eating. This postural shift helps food move faster to the duodenum, resulting in increased CCK levels and a nearly immediate reduction in hunger.

Corticotrophin: Corticotrophin is the neurotransmitter released in response to stress. Stress-induced corticotrophin inhibits the effectiveness of the digestive system and can reduce the desire for food in some individuals. This connection between high-stress levels and poor digestion is not coincidental. However, it's important to highlight that a balanced breakfast can serve as a powerful defense mechanism against eating disorders and binge eating, especially for individuals with demanding daily routines.

Dopamine, Adrenaline, and Noradrenaline: These neurotransmitters, often referred to as the "feel-good" chemicals, provide a sense of control, efficacy, and alertness. They have a direct influence on mental states and assist in the production of thyroid hormones. These neurotransmitters are synthesized from amino acids like tyrosine and phenylalanine found in protein-rich foods such as meat, fish, beans, nuts, seeds, soybeans, and cheese. A deficiency of these foods in one's daily diet can significantly affect hunger and satiety mechanisms.

Endorphins: Endorphins are a group of powerful brain and body substances that enhance satisfaction and pleasure while also increasing pain tolerance. They are often described as "our personal opioids." Endorphins are capable of inducing pleasure and reducing pain, making them responsible for various forms of euphoria, joy, heightened self-esteem, and enjoyment. Low levels of endorphins can increase appetite and might be due to factors like genetics, stress, and gender diversity. Increased endorphin levels can occur through activities like deep breathing, exercise, and dietary choices. The adequate intake of specific vitamins (B, D, C), minerals (magnesium, calcium), and essential fatty acids (EFAs) is crucial for maintaining satisfactory endorphin levels.

A balanced and nutritious diet rich in high-protein foods, fresh vegetables, and essential fatty acids can support endorphin production. In contrast, low-fat and highly caloric restrictive diets can deplete endorphin reserves, notably if they lack protein and fat. Certain foods, like chocolate and sugar, contain opioid peptides due to incomplete digestion, potentially contributing to low endorphin levels. Consuming such foods repetitively can create a dependency relationship. Proper nutrition and maintaining satisfactory levels of endorphins are vital for overall well-being and appetite control.

In conclusion, the intricate web of neurotransmitters and their impact on appetite, mood, and overall health underscores the complexity of human biology. A thorough understanding of the role of these chemicals, as well as the influence of diet, digestion, and stress, is essential for promoting a balanced, healthy approach to eating and mental well-being.

Serotonin: Serotonin, a neurotransmitter, plays a multifaceted role in our bodies, influencing various aspects of our health. It is essential for transmitting critical messages between cells and is primarily found in the gastrointestinal tract, where it regulates stomach acids, digestive juices, and bowel movements. An insufficiency of serotonin production can lead to issues such as constipation and gastroesophageal reflux disease. Yet, its most well-known function revolves around brain chemistry. Serotonin is associated with numerous critical functions in the body, ensuring smooth nerve signal transmission and circulation.

Within the brain, large clusters of serotonin-producing neurons are distributed throughout various regions. It is believed that there are more than fifteen distinct types of serotonin receptors, each playing a unique role in different bodily functions. Additionally, serotonin acts as a chemical regulator, influencing the balance of various neurotransmitters. The significance of serotonin in maintaining mental health has led to the development of several serotonergic synthetic drugs, with Prozac and Ladoz being among the most commonly used for treating depression.

2.1.17 The Impact of Serotonin on the Brain

Serotonin exerts its influence on mood, the perception of pain, sexual behavior, and sleep, but its most pivotal role lies in controlling appetite through the mechanism of "fullness and satiation." It acts as a brake on food intake by sending specific signals to the brain, indicating that sufficient food has been consumed.

Serotonin cannot be ingested directly from external sources and reach the brain; instead, it is synthesized from the essential amino acid tryptophan. Tryptophan is converted into 5HPP and further transformed into serotonin through enzymatic processes. This process requires several nutritional factors, including B vitamins, magnesium, iron, and chromium.

Tryptophan, the major precursor of serotonin, is naturally found in various foods, including milk, oatmeal, legumes, poultry, eggs, red meat, soybeans, yogurt, nuts, sesame seeds, tahini, and more. Consuming a wide variety of these foods in your daily diet is essential to ensure an adequate intake of tryptophan and maintain serotonin levels. Diets that are lacking in nutrients or monotonous in nature can significantly disrupt the balance of the human body.

Interestingly, carbohydrates play a role in increasing serotonin levels due to their ability to enhance tryptophan absorption. Even chocolate, known for its rich tryptophan content, can lead to dependence in individuals. This dependency, however, seems to be linked to chocolates that contain milk, possibly due to the casein amino acid present in milk. Casein competes with tryptophan for access to the brain, potentially explaining the craving for milk chocolate. Consuming small quantities of dark chocolate, typically around 10-30 grams, without inducing addiction, may be related to its combination with almonds or hazelnuts, or pairing it with uncooked unsalted nuts. This balanced approach offers a satisfying and pleasurable snack while keeping daily calorie intake in check.

Moreover, foods like avocado, pineapple, bananas, plums, and tomatoes are natural sources of serotonin.

2.1.18 Serotonin Deficiency and Bulimia

Why do many individuals experience serotonin deficiency, and how does it relate to conditions like bulimia?

An imbalance in brain chemistry is a situation that can be expected to some extent due to modern life's stressors and lifestyle factors. Most people's diets lack essential nutrients, depriving their bodies of the raw materials needed to produce sufficient serotonin. Factors such as fatigue, emotional stress, and poor eating habits can force the body to continually adapt to maintain chemical balance, which is constantly disrupted due to stress depleting essential nutrients. These factors can rapidly decrease the brain's ability to produce adequate serotonin to meet the body's daily requirements. Furthermore, serotonin cannot be externally administered to the brain; it can only be produced internally.

Lack of tryptophan, low serotonin, and eating disorders create a complex interplay. Tryptophan must compete with other amino acids to access the brain. When a protein-rich diet is consumed, tryptophan often loses the competition due to its minimal presence in foods. On the other hand, when carbohydrates are ingested along with protein, insulin release prevents several competing amino acids, allowing tryptophan to cross into the brain and produce serotonin.

2.1.19 The Connection between Carbohydrates and Serotonin Deficiency

A strong desire for carbohydrates might be linked to serotonin deficiency. As serotonin levels decrease, various complications like depression, obesity, insomnia, migraines, chronic fatigue, premenstrual syndrome, and Seasonal Affective Disorder (SAD) can emerge. SAD is characterized by mood disturbances during specific periods, typically in the winter, leading to symptoms often referred to as "winter depression." The most common feature in all these situations is binge-eating episodes, mainly focused on carbohydrates.

Studies have revealed that when individuals, both humans and animals, are on tryptophan-deficient diets, their appetite increases in proportion to serotonin levels. However, long-term hypocaloric and low food intake diets can decrease serotonin and tryptophan levels in the blood. Since serotonin plays a critical role in appetite regulation, low serotonin levels can trigger bulimic episodes characterized by the consumption of large quantities of food, particularly foods rich in simple carbohydrates like sugar and starch.

2.1.20 The Vicious Cycle of Bulimia and Carbohydrate Binge-Eating Episodes

Binge-eating episodes, especially involving carbohydrate-rich foods, provide a quick energy source for the body.

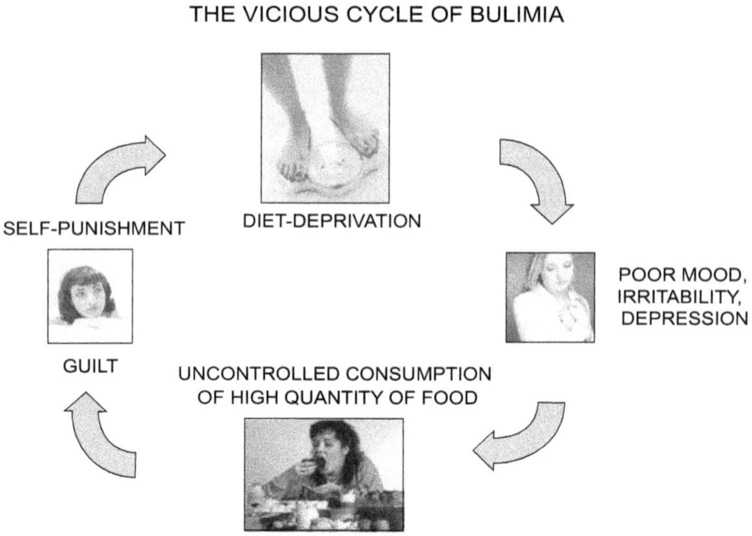

THE VICIOUS CYCLE OF BULIMIA

DIET-DEPRIVATION

POOR MOOD, IRRITABILITY, DEPRESSION

UNCONTROLLED CONSUMPTION OF HIGH QUANTITY OF FOOD

GUILT

SELF-PUNISHMENT

Figure 2.1 The vicious cycle of bulimia.

2.2 The Importance of a Properly Selected Nutrition Plan

2.2.1 Hyperphagia and Protein Adequacy: A Key to Managing Binge Eating

Many individuals are particularly susceptible to binge eating episodes during the evening and night. Incorporating protein into each meal and snack can help maintain stable blood glucose levels and ensure adequate tryptophan intake through the diet. Research indicates that when protein content falls below 5% in a meal, the brain's absorption of tryptophan is hindered. An ideal daily protein intake should be at least 100 grams, distributed across various meals. Those who tend to experience binge eating episodes at night may benefit from consuming a substantial amount of protein during dinner.

2.2.2 Light Exposure and Serotonin-Melatonin Balance

Light plays a crucial role in regulating the balance between serotonin and melatonin in our bodies. Darkness signals the pineal gland to convert serotonin into melatonin, which induces sleep. Bright light disrupts this process, preventing the conversion. People residing in areas with insufficient lighting are at risk of melatonin overload and serotonin deficiency. To maintain optimal serotonin levels, meals should be enjoyed under bright light, never in low-light conditions. In the treatment of eating disorders, it's important to ensure daily sun exposure of at least 30 minutes, particularly during peak sunshine hours.

2.2.3 The Importance of Snacking to Manage Binge Eating

Snacking is essential for effectively managing binge eating episodes. The key rule is to have a snack or a meal rich in complex carbohydrates when an individual is most likely to experience a binge eating episode, allowing the tryptophan pathway to open on time. A meal or snack rich in complex carbohydrates can boost serotonin levels for approximately three hours, while a protein-based meal can inhibit the brain's tryptophan recovery for at least two hours. It's critical that these carbohydrates come from complex, unprocessed sources to prevent undesirable hypoglycemia. Foods like fruit or natural juices, paired with high-fiber snacks, offer a suitable solution. Otherwise, hypoglycemia can exacerbate serotonin deficiency symptoms and contribute to unnecessary weight gain.

2.2.4 5-HTP: A Natural Precursor of Serotonin

5-HTP is a natural amino acid compound extracted from the seeds of the Griffonia plant and Valerian root. It is used in the brain to produce serotonin and has been a dietary supplement for the treatment of depression, sleep disorders, obesity, and various other conditions for decades. 5-HTP is more fat-soluble than tryptophan and closely resembles serotonin's structure in the brain. It can cross the blood-brain barrier without the need for a transport protein, allowing for rapid and immediate action. Using 5-HTP does not disrupt insulin secretion. By increasing serotonin levels, 5-HTP positively affects the mechanisms of satiety and can help control daily caloric intake. Additionally, improved mood and increased energy levels make adhering to a diet and exercise plan more manageable. Extensive research on 5-HTP as a treatment agent has not been associated with severe adverse reactions, except in cases of overdose leading to nausea. Moreover, it has not been linked to dependence.

2.2.5 5-HTP and Sleep Quality

5-HTP influences all monoamine neurotransmitters, including dopamine and noradrenaline, which counteract the effects of melatonin, a hormone produced by serotonin that induces sleep. Melatonin is primarily released during the night, even when serotonin levels are higher. The use of 5-HTP as a dietary supplement should be supervised by a specialized nutritionist or therapist. It should never be combined with St. John's Wort or SSRI treatment.

2.2.6 Nutritional Factors Essential for Serotonin Production and Balance

Various nutritional factors are required for the synthesis and administration of serotonin, including:

- B vitamins, especially B1, B5, B6, B12, and folic acid
- Magnesium
- Vitamin C
- Chromium (for insulin production)
- Other Factors Affecting Serotonin Levels

Exercise: Engaging in regular exercise helps burn calories, reduce stress and anxiety, enhance mood, and boost self-esteem. It can also help prevent overindulgence in carbohydrates and alcohol.

Stress Control: Teaching individuals with eating disorders to manage stress through cognitive and behavioral techniques can help maintain consistent nutrient levels, using quality food sources.

Neuropeptide Y: Stress, fear, and anger can elevate neuropeptide Y levels, impacting serotonin secretion and leading to increased carbohydrate consumption. Long or short intervals between meals can also affect neuropeptide Y levels, intensifying feelings of hunger. Establishing a regular meal schedule is key to managing neuropeptide Y levels. Additionally, mild exercise with a duration of about one hour requires a small carbohydrate snack before and after exercise to maintain neuropeptide Y levels at an optimum level.

Limitation of Sweeteners: Various sweeteners used in products like chewing gum, sugar substitutes, and dietetic formulas, especially when combined with caffeine, can act as powerful stimulants. Aspartame can block tryptophan metabolism, hindering serotonin production. Additionally, these products create confusion in the body's hunger and satiety mechanisms, leading to overconsumption.

2.2.7 Conclusion

The overstimulation of neurotransmitter receptors over time has contributed to the development of dependency on substances like chocolate and sweets. This overstimulation has led to the body's need for increasing doses of these substances to achieve the desired effects like euphoria, satisfaction, and happiness. This is due to the brain's dependence on escalating doses of the substance to maintain neurotransmitter levels.

2.2.8 The Importance of a Well-Designed Diet

A well-designed diet plan is essential for individuals suffering from eating disorders to restore their body's biochemical balance gradually. A diet characterized by variety, harmony, and the appropriate combination of nutrient-rich foods can address various problems caused by malnutrition, low energy, weakened body strength, constipation, and more. Timely, consistent meals at intervals of two to three hours can help avoid hypoglycemia symptoms and ensure a steady nutrient supply.

2.2.9 The Significance of Fluid Intake

Inadequate fluid intake can have numerous adverse effects on health. Dehydration is a widespread issue, affecting around 75% of Americans. Furthermore, approximately 37% of Americans have such a weak thirst mechanism that it is often confused with hunger. Therefore, the importance of staying hydrated cannot be overstated. Consuming a glass of water shortly before bedtime can alleviate nighttime hunger or midnight cravings for nearly 100% of individuals. Moreover, even mild dehydration can reduce metabolism by at least 3%, affecting energy levels. Proper hydration throughout the day is essential for overall health.

2.3 The Importance of Adequate Sleep for Hunger and Satiation Mechanisms

2.3.1 The Association of Sleep with a Healthy Weight

There is a direct correlation between the quality of sleep and the variability of body weight. Poor sleep quality can result in difficulty losing weight, a decrease in metabolism and a disruption in the functioning of hormones. In addition, sleep deprivation has been associated with the occurrence of pathological conditions such as type 2 diabetes mellitus, hypertension and cardiovascular disease.

Through a study carried out by myself and my colleagues entitled "Sleep Deprivation: Effects on Weight Loss and Weight Loss Maintenance", 1054 studies were examined with the goal to investigate the important role the quality sleep plays in weight loss. Studying the research findings, it was observed that the circadian rhythm/clock was a major contributor in improving body weight and in the orderly functioning of the body.

2.3.2 The Importance of Sleep in Changing and Maintaining Body Weight

Through the literature research carried out, it was found that sleep affects the reduction or maintenance of body weight. In particular, it appeared that people who had quality sleep of more than 7 hours showcased better management of their body weight. On the contrary, people who did not follow 7 hours of sleep, combined with its poor quality, showed difficulty maintaining or reducing their body weight. People who achieved weight loss of 5% or more appeared to have better sleep quality at night. Finally, a shift from fat oxidation to carbohydrate oxidation was observed.

2.3.3 Diet and Sleep

As it was seen, sleep is affected by the composition of the diet and vice versa. Thus, people who followed a strict 800-calorie diet had poor-quality sleep. In particular, poor quality sleep means that during this process the body did not perform slow wave sleep (SWS), which means they did not sleep ¨heavily¨. In addition, short sleep duration is related to energy intake and the type of food consumed during the day. So, people who had consumed a large amount of sugar or sugar-free carbohydrates showed nocturnal hyperarousal. Also, foods high in saturated fat and foods low in fiber, i.e., avoiding fruits and vegetables, have been associated with poor quality sleep. It was much easier for people who got 8.5 hours of sleep to reduce their body fat percentage than people who only got 5.5 hours of sleep.

2.3.4 Sleep and Hormones

The circadian rhythm, which is a biological process of the body, plays an important role in sleep management. It is affected by external factors, such as sunlight and temperature changes. So, when our bodily functions are harmonized with its circadian rhythm, the metabolic processes and the functioning of the hormones are regulated accordingly. Some hormones increase or decrease the feeling of hunger and satiety.

So, the studies showed that sleep of poor quality and in disharmony with the body's circadian rhythm, can disrupt the functioning of these hormones. The result of this disorder is that these hormones become either overactive or underactive. In more detail, the study showed that leptin, the hormone responsible for satiety and correspondingly for the metabolic processes related to the utilization of energy, is regulated while the subject receives adequate sleep, while its function is deceased during sleep deprivation periods, making weight loss difficult. On the contrary, the secretion of the hormones ghrelin and cortisol, which regulate hunger and stress respectively, increase when sleep is not of good quality.

2.3.5 Conclusion

As a result of the analysis we carried out, the crucial importance of sleep was confirmed, as it acts multifactorially. Sleep quality has a direct impact on reducing or maintaining body weight. Finally, quality sleep regulates the hormonal system to function properly, with the physical signals of hunger and satiety functioning in harmony making for better body weight management.

2.3.6 Things to Do 60 Minutes before Going to Bed

- Under no circumstances should you lie in bed before the time that you want to sleep in, unless you have more pleasant plans in mind.
- Turn off all electronic devices that emit blue light.
- Instead of exchanging a stream of messages, and thus continuously exposing yourself to blue light, try calling the person with whom you are communicating. This will also allow you to have more personal communication.
- If you watch television one hour before bedtime, try reading a book instead which is more pleasant. Avoid stories that may stress or trouble you. The ideal position would be sitting in an armchair with light coming from a reading lamp positioned behind your head and to the left. Reading is made much more pleasant this way.
- Turn on the radio or put on a relaxing playlist. I frequently reminisce about the days of late-night radio shows with their numerous song requests!
- Wash your teeth immediately after dinner. This has two advantages: it will discourage any attempt of late-night snacking and you will not have to turn on the bright bathroom lights, and thus disrupt the production of melatonin, to brush your teeth before going to bed.

- Wear your pyjamas, or comfortable clothes that are not tight on your body, especially the area around the stomach. It has been found that when a person has dinner wearing clothes that are tight in the stomach area, they increase the chances of indigestion and acid flux during the night.
- Turn off or dim all lights that are too intense in the room.
- If you need to do something that requires turning on the light, use the flashlight of your smartphone or a similarly dimmer source of light.
- Even if your sleep is interrupted, for example to go to the bathroom, again use a dim source of light to navigate your way.
- Avoid any conversation that may disturb you in any manner during the hours of the evening. Another recommendation I will give you is to "never make an important decision before a good night's rest". You really can't go wrong following this advice.
- If you feel drowsy while sitting in the sofa or armchair, it is probably a good time to go to bed. If you let yourself nap there, it will be very difficult to go into deep sleep when you go to bed later, as your body will have received a short boost of energy that will negatively affect the production of melatonin.
- Consumption of liquids and especially alcoholic beverages of all kinds should be avoided.
- Consumption of coffee (even decaf) or caffeinated beverages should also be avoided for at least 6 hours before going to bed.
- Finally, before closing your eyes you should take the time to express your gratitude for at least 3 good things that happened to you and thanking those who did something good for you. For example, you could thank the polite man who let me pass in front of him that morning that you were in a hurry, thank your friend that called to see how I was doing instead of just sending a lifeless message.

It is thus as important that you follow a steady sleep schedule as it is to keep to a specific meal plan. Your biological clock is set to set off hunger at specific times so that you can avoid unnecessary snacking all the time. Falling asleep will also become easier when your body is scheduled to go into "sleep mode" at regular hours. The more you get a regular and good quality sleep, the better you will be able to manage the quantity and quality of your meals during the day.

2.4 Summary

Gathering data for the second chapter each day during my research for this book, I noticed that advertising and promoting the wonders of surgical treatment of obesity by the media was continually increasing. Coincidentally, I was invited to a corresponding program on surgical obesity. I found that what took place was the presentation of these surgeries as the absolute miracle of bariatrics, as it is commonly called scientifically. However, a vigilant viewer would quickly find that treated patients present, who reported losing weight, rarely remained in this condition for more than 12-18 months post-surgery. And finally, for some mysterious reason, of all those overweight individuals who had lost 50 to 80 pounds, everyone had stopped at 44-66 pounds over their normal weight, and no one looked like a normally weighing person. When it came time to present the results of two very thin women who had undergone surgery five years before, I found that the first one was only 53 years old, her face looking like she was 80, and the second was so skinny, her body weight was way within the range of anorexia.

Since an ancient Greek saying says that "you need to be intelligent to understand that you are a fool," I would like to ask one question to everyone. As, apart from having no more room for food in the stomach, there are many other mechanisms that can lead to a restriction on food intake, why should anyone opt for the surgeon's table? Because all these experts say that the problem of obese people will be solved magically, it is to just a matter of putting them under the knife or incapacitating - bypassing their stomach or intestines. Because they never bothered to explain to their prospective clients that the problem is not just how to fill the stomach or not (since there will be no stomach post-surgery), but the myriad of side effects that follow. How is it possible for prominent scientists to apply the most unorthodox technique according to Hippocrates of "cutting the hand that hurts" when after surgery the cut stomach or intestine has been lost forever, leaving a series of incredible complications for the future? All health experts know that rapid weight loss not only represents a reduction in unnecessary body fat but also, to a great extent, muscle and tissue degradation of the whole body which in the next 4-5 years will lead to the complete physical weakening as well as a reduction of life expectancy. And what image will this body present after abrupt slimming? The skin will teem with scars like an elderly person, a female breast will sag 'till the belly and the belly 'till the knees. Clearly, plastic surgeries will follow, but who guarantees they will have a positive result? They will certainly be numerous. Also, how much will these plastic surgeries cost, and who will pay for them?

And if, based on evidence that more than 50,000 such operations have taken place in Greece in the past 10 years, where are all these happy, slim people? Why are there no statistics whatsoever about what has happened? Where are all those who have undergone similar interventions after 5 or 6 years? Do they live among us? Does the homonymous popular film by John Carpenter refer to them?

Obese people clearly also have a reduced life expectancy, but before the surgery, why were they never presented with the choice to improve their diet and exercise? "For every 1 hour of daily walking, one gains 1 day of life" as we say in my cycle. If you are 40 and live your life as an overweight individual, you will live up to 50 because, statistically, you will have a heart attack and pray you are not on vacation on a barren island because no one will be able to save you. But, if you walk for 1 hour and eat properly, instead of 50, you will reach 60, and if you do that until 60 you will reach 80. I won't even mention the psychological disorders all these people will be led to since the limited amount of food their disturbed digestive system will manage to utilize, will not be enough to regulate any of the chemicals and neurotransmitters required for the chemical balance of the brain. I've really wondered many times whether the "obesity surgeons" themselves are aware of the existence of all these other factors that regulate hunger beyond the stomach itself. I would like to close this section by quoting the phrase of a lady who once visited me after a similar operation: "Before surgery, I was a happy obese person. Now after the surgery, I am an unhappy obese person."

2.5 Key Takeaways

1. **Hunger and Satiety Mechanisms:**
    - Hunger and satiety are natural processes regulating food intake.
    - Imbalances in these processes can lead to overeating or insufficient nutrient consumption.
2. **The Role of Serotonin:**
    - Serotonin affects appetite and food choices, especially during stressful situations.
    - Increasing serotonin through proper nutrition and physical activity helps stabilize mood.
3. **The Role of Glucose:**
    - Blood glucose levels influence hunger; managing these levels can improve the relationship with food.
    - Sharp fluctuations in glucose are linked to intense hunger and unhealthy food cravings.
4. **The Impact of Sleep:**
    - Insufficient sleep affects levels of hormones regulating appetite, increasing the risk of overeating.
    - Maintaining a consistent sleep cycle helps with better dietary management.
5. **The Psychological Factor:**
    - Emotional trauma and stress can significantly influence eating behaviours.
    - Strengthening self-esteem and developing emotional regulation can support recovery from eating disorders.
6. **Nutritional Education:**
    - Learning to choose high-nutritional-value foods can restore natural hunger-satiety mechanisms.
    - Planning balanced meals with adequate nutrients is crucial for long-term health.

Chapter 3

Training People with Eating Disorders

A large belly may bear unrealised ideas and desires.
Until they are realized... it grows.

3.1 Training in Simple Terms

3.1.1 The Importance of Training Patients with an Eating Disorder

At first, being trained on and understanding the mechanisms of glucose and serotonin should be seen as an integral part of the education and information every client who asks for our help in losing weight should receive. Experience has shown that it is the only way to motivate the client to adopt better eating habits. It is also very important that this training be carried out in a comprehensible and straightforward manner without any scientific terms; this way, the client can immediately understand both its importance and how proper nutrition works. Some simple examples of how all these biochemical functions can be made more comprehensive are shown below.

We often find that not everyone is always ready to go on a weight-loss program, so we still explain that it is imperative before the diet that normal hunger and satiety mechanisms be restored. As far as the factors of stress and customer readiness, this is something we

Nutritional Intelligence: The Answer to Bulimia, Overeating, and Obesity
Evangelos Zoumbaneas

ISBN 978-981-5129-74-8 (Hardcover), 978-981-5129-73-1 (Paperback), 978-1-003-65188-8 (eBook)
www.jennystanford.com

should continuously review. Some clients often realize that they may not be ready to follow a diet; however, through education, they recognize that it is essential to stop causing more harm to themselves by gaining more weight because they simply cannot start losing it at a certain point in time. So, they learn that they can take care of themselves nutritionally whether they are in a maintenance, or weight loss period or in a diet phase.

3.1.2 A Properly Chosen Diet Plan as the First Step of Treatment

It is imperative, now, to return to an earlier normal state where every living being, whether human or animal, knows precisely how much it needs to eat, avoiding consumption of excess food beyond satiation. As I have mentioned many times, in nature there are hardly any obese animals apart from those of the human species. We will never meet any animal exceeding the needs that nature itself has set for it to always have the ideal fat and body weight ratio. Experiments performed on animals and especially mice, in which they stopped receiving fresh foods such as fruits, vegetables and fruits and were instead fed with processed, manufactured foods such as potato chips, biscuits and white flour they soon lost control of eating and consequently nearly doubled their daily calorie intake and became overweight. When they replaced their food again with natural foods, the normal hunger and satiety mechanisms soon returned to their normal function and later they gradually went back to their original weight before the start of the experiment.

Restoring people's natural mechanisms of hunger and saturation that nature intended them to have as a primordial instinct to ensure a permanent balance between themselves and their environment is or great importance. This primitive instinct that young children have determining when they have had enough, ceasing eating even if the most delicious food is available. It is an inner natural instinct, a primordial internal mechanism that is best preserved as long as the foods consumed are closer to their natural form. That is, the foods we offer our body need to be as fresh as possible, and less processed. The answer to modern people's inability to control the amount of food they consume comes through the food itself. After first collecting all the necessary nutrients they need to ensure their body's smooth function, they can then supply it with whatever else they want. Let us follow the example mentioned in Chapter 1 with the diet of two halves. Preventing binge eating episodes is of primary importance due to lack of all necessary nutrients and addressing the psychological causes that lead to over-eating can be handled at a later point. A properly chosen diet will be similar to first aid to a severely injured person. It is like the ambulance that will arrive at the scene of the accident in time. After the first aid is provided, they will keep him alive until hospitalization. It's like a body with multiple bleeding wounds. First, we have to treat them and then proceed to mending and restoration of the wounds. This is precisely how the restoration of a properly selected and adequate nutrition works for people suffering from any form of an eating disorder. It is the duty of all health practitioners, especially of dietitians, to first reconstitute the body's physiological mechanisms and then leave those who are familiar with the origins of eating disorders cure the causes that led to this disorganization. Seeking a suitable psychotherapist will then be crucial to preventing the patient from relapsing. Without treatment of all the reasons that led to binge eating, the risk will always be visible, and it will be just a matter of time until it worsens again. A deterioration that will always lead the unfortunate patient to a worse condition than the one they were in until a little time before. For a person already suffering from an eating disorder, diet and hypocaloric nutrition will lead with mathematical precision to further deterioration. Any recent relapse will lead to an even more significant loss of physical and mental health until psychiatric treatment appears to be the only way out. Please mark the words I use: "Psychiatric" treatment as the only means of a "possible" recovery.

3.1.3 The Explanation of Serotonin Synthesis in the Brain

Every time we eat protein food such as meat, fish, egg, dairy, etc., it breaks down in the body into all the individual proteins it is made up of.

For example, remember the last time you had a piece of beef and remember cutting it with a knife.

You would notice that it consists of many fibres attached to each other. Suppose each of these fibres is a single protein.

If we could isolate and magnify this fibre-protein, we would see that it is made up of other small beads called amino acids.

Each of these beads is also an amino acid.

One of these amino acids is called tryptophan (T-shaped pellet).

When released into the blood, Tryptophan can go through a specific carrier to enter the brain and then convert to another substance called serotonin (Figure 3.1).

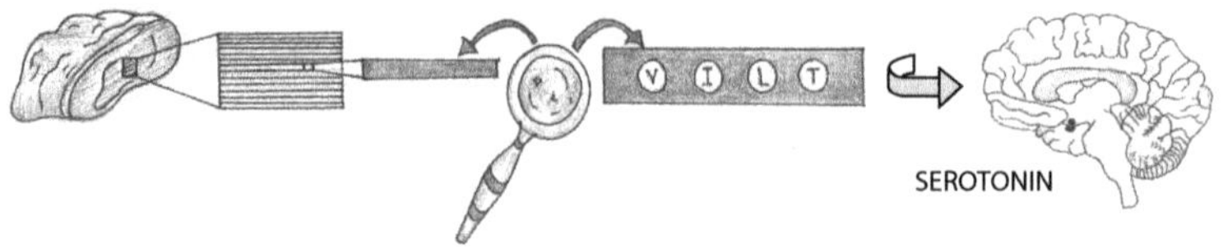

Figure 3.1

Serotonin is a substance that, when formed in the brain, creates a sense of satiety. That is, it has a positive effect on our mood. For example, our attitude towards a cloudy day can either be positive or negative and this is relative to serotonin. Whether we hit the horn immediately after the traffic light turns green and begin screaming and yelling at the driver in front of us, or we choose to wait patiently for the traffic to start rolling, has got to do with serotonin. Whether we slowly eat a serving of food or greedily devour it, has to do with serotonin. Simply put, serotonin affects our mood and ability to stop eating once we have consumed a serving of food.

If we consume a serving of protein, we will receive a sufficient amount of tryptophan. Then an adequate amount of serotonin will be produced, thus giving us this sense of satiation.

And if we manage to do this three times during a day, that is, in the morning, noon, and evening, our day will generally be better, and we will consume precisely as much food as we need without desire to eat anything more.

So, the issue of good mood and hunger would simply be solved if we could consume a serving of protein each morning, noon, and evening. For example, this would work if we had a glass of milk at breakfast, a serving of chicken at lunch, and one of cheese at dinner.

But as we have mentioned above, every protein fibre contains other amino acids, apart from that of tryptophan, with equally bizarre names such as valine (V bead), leucine (L bead), isoleucine (I bead); besides the oddity of their names, they also are more likely to compete with tryptophan (T), to displace it and eventually prevent it from entering the brain (Figure 3.2). The result is that almost no serotonin is created.

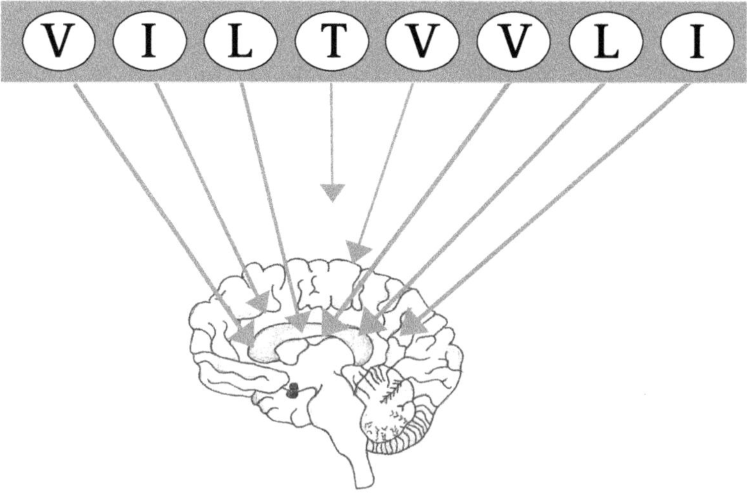

Figure 3.2 In the figure, we see that all amino acids claim a position to pass to the brain, pushing tryptophan out.

If we add a serving of starch to a serving of protein, then the body will have the pancreas secrete insulin to digest the starch. Insulin takes all amino-acids, other than tryptophan, to the various tissues where they will be used to restore other damaged tissues. I remind you that exercising aids in this. This way tryptophan will be left undisturbed to enter the brain and create the much-needed serotonin. For example, this issue would be solved if we added a serving of cereals or a couple of slices of bread or toast, or if we added a serving of rice or potato to our lunch and ate a wholegrain rusk with our evening serving of cheese.

If alongside these foods, we added one more that contains vitamin C such as fruit at breakfast, a salad at lunch or a little grated tomato in the evening to make a nice "Dacos" salad (Greek salad with barley rusk, grated tomatoes and feta cheese) then the process of serotonin production would take place very quickly since vitamin C itself can expedite this process.

In Figure 3.3, we see that after eating a starch-containing meal, the pancreas produces insulin, and it, in turn, sends amino acids V, I, and L to the muscles and various organs leaving tryptophan (T) free to enter the brain to produce serotonin.

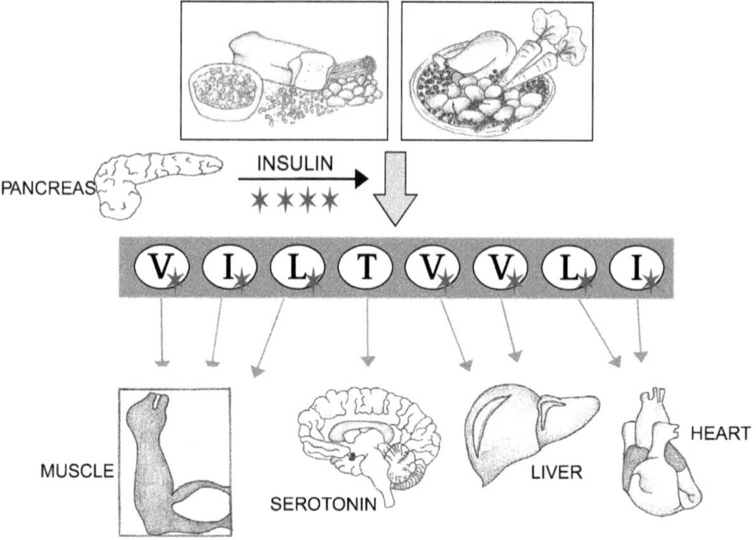

Figure 3.3 In the figure, we see that after eating a starch-containing meal, the pancreas produces insulin, and it, in turn, sends amino acids V, I, and L to the muscles and various organs leaving tryptophan (T) free to enter the brain to produce serotonin.

Here lies the miracle of the traditional Greek diet: all meals are combined to produce serotonin continuously.

For example, eat baked meat (protein) with potatoes (starch) and combine it with salad (vitamin C).

We eat green beans (vitamin C), cook them with potatoes (starch) and combine them with feta cheese (protein).

We cook beans (starch and protein together). In the same pan, we add carrots, celery, onions (vitamin C) and combine them with feta cheese (protein).

We cook meat (protein), garnish it with rice (starch), and combine it with salad (vitamin C).

We grate fresh tomatoes (vitamin C), garnish with grated feta cheese (protein), put them on a rusk (starch) and make a tasty Cretan Dakos.

We cut tomato, cucumber, peppers, onion (vitamin C), add a piece of feta cheese (protein), and make a Greek salad to combine with a slice of baked bread (starch).

And supposing we add a little extra virgin olive oil to all of these foods, the good fats will help the brain cells (mainly made of fat) remain healthy and always able to allow all these strange chemical reactions which are so beneficial to our mental and physical well-being to take place easily.

Thus, it is of paramount importance that every meal we have consists of foods from all three essential groups, that is, a serving of fruits or vegetables with a serving of protein and one of starch to ensure an adequate quantity of serotonin for the brain. These "magic" food triads that we will see later in various alternative combinations are completely responsible for our psychological well-being but also our ability to consume exactly the amount of food we need.

3.1.4 The Explanation of the Mechanism of Glucose

The carbohydrates from our food, mainly from sweet and starchy foods, are absorbed by the intestine in the form of glucose. After being absorbed by the intestine, glucose passes into the bloodstream and is then transferred to the cells to immediately produce the necessary energy. Blood contains about 20g of glucose, which is depleted within a few hours, as the body's cells use it to continuously produce energy. A significant serving of this amount of glucose is continuously used by brain cells. In particular, one-third of our energy needs correspond to the function of the brain. The brain seeks to maintain its constant glucose supply at any cost, even if the amount of consumed calories is far greater than what is necessary. The brain contains glucose detectors found in the hypothalamus and affect the supply of any amount of glucose absorbed by the cells. If we don't consume food for many hours and glucose levels fall, the first thing affected is our sound judgment, that is, the proper decisions made by the brain. A typical example is that people who have not had food for a long period of time, cannot later control the amount of food they consume.

Blood glucose levels and the way glucose levels are recognized by the brain are determined by the' hormone insulin, secreted in the pancreas when consuming carbohydrates. The role of insulin is to transport glucose to the body's cells, where it acts on the muscle cell receptors. Every muscle and tissue cell, such as the heart or brain, is like a miniature factory that burns glucose to produce energy. And the point is not that cells burn glucose at some random point to produce energy, but that they burn and use glucose constantly, even when we are asleep. So, it is easy to see how volatile this organism's fuel can be and how important it is to regularly replenish blood glucose reserves.

For this reason, as soon as blood glucose levels drop, the hunger mechanism automatically starts to initiate the process of finding food. Suppose energy requirements for carbohydrates are not met immediately - about 2-2.5 hours after the last meal - glucose stores will be depleted. In that case, blood levels will be too low, and there is a high chance of hypoglycaemia. The symptoms of prolonged hypoglycaemia are tachycardia, sweating, dizziness, hunger, weakness, fatigue, blurred vision, confusion, and the worse thing is that without us realizing, all the factors that lead to stress increase. Under these conditions and due to stress created in the body, the most common reaction to hypoglycaemia is to consume huge amounts of food and especially those high in starch, sugar, and calories such as cookies, sweets, chocolates, chocolates, soft drinks with sugar, chocolate milk, etc.

Also, when these foods are consumed, blood glucose levels rise and then, having absorbed the amount of glucose it needs all at once, the body cannot manage the rest and leaves it in the blood. Then all the unused amount of glucose in the blood is transferred by insulin again, only this time, it is unfortunately taken for storage in fat cells. The body will immediately utilize the amount of glucose it needs to rapidly nourish the body and brain cells and turn the rest into fat (Figure 3.4).

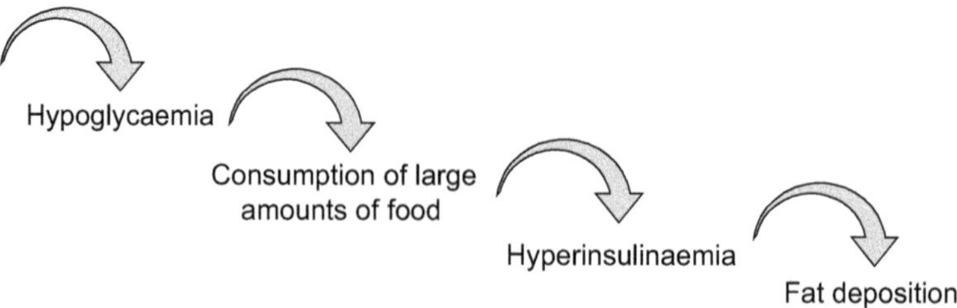

Figure 3.4

This way, when the time for a meal comes, even if a person has the strongest will, they will not be able to stop eating more than he or she needs, because due to hypoglycaemia the brain is unable of resisting. There is no way to make the right choices e.g., starting their meal with salad because "the body turns into a beast thirsty not for blood, but for carbohydrates" and will start with foods like potatoes, bread, spaghetti that will satisfy its hunger instincts. When the blood glucose balance returns after 20-30 minutes, all the brain can do is realize its mistake and regret the consumption of what has already been eaten on the promise that it will not happen again. And unfortunately, it will happen again. Figures 3.5 and 3.6 are schematic representations of what is mentioned in the following paragraph.

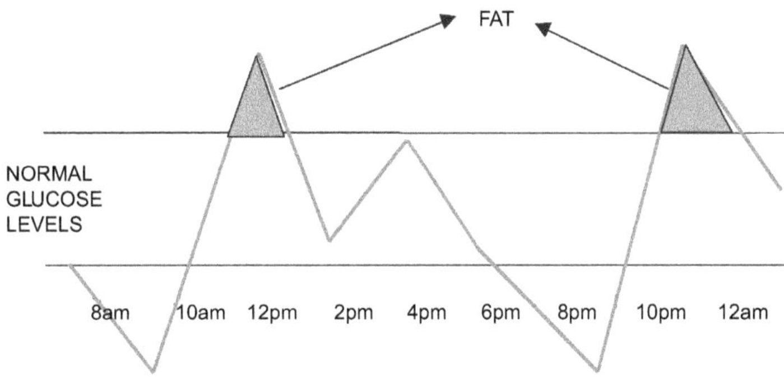

Figure 3.5

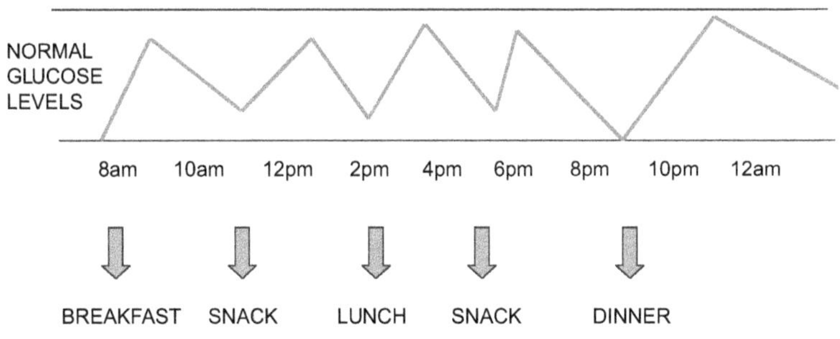

Figure 3.6

One of the biggest mistakes people make in their diet is "foolish self-esteem". They believe that if they avoid almost all of the intermediate snacks and eat a single meal, then they will lose weight. The classic statement "I will not eat anything all day in order to eat more at night." also belongs in this behavioural category. These tactics are exactly what we need to follow if we wish to completely deregulate the brain's natural biochemical processes that determine the mechanisms of hunger and satiety. The answer to this is to make sure we eat small and properly combined meals whose nutrients will then be coded and transformed into "key compounds" that literally "lock hunger". Unfortunately, those who suffer from eating disorders either remain without food for long periods of time or the foods they choose are nutrient- deficient, meaning they do not contain the right "keys" to help them cope with the difficult times a bulimic crisis is at the gates. Even if one manages to control the amount of food they eat by making the wrong choices, there is no way this incorrect way of control will last longer than two months. Two months is a milestone for anyone dieting, when their diet is limited in calories without their minding the nutritional content and right combination of meals. Typical examples are calorie-based, protein or monophagia diets. Two months is the maximum time any human body can withstand, followed by breaking of the diet and the prompt return to a weight greater to that before the beginning of the diet. With this tactic, the diet "veteran" interrupts the diet every two months, changes his diet, or once again discovers some new magic slimming method. This has nothing to do with the lack of willpower but the disorganisation of the body's natural defence mechanisms. It has nothing to do with the fact that after two months there was probably not enough motivation, but the lack of the magic keys that would lock the beast of bulimia back to its cage. The beast will always be there, every day and hour. Every moment when a critical meal has been skipped, it lingers behind your back, waiting for your first moment of weakness to devour you. If bulimia is treated thoughtlessly, if a person doesn't learn how to deal with it and doesn't understand the mechanisms and the techniques required for him to be able to tame it, then it is probably going to grow old with him, and the person will end up spending his life trying different unsuccessful diets. The more the diets, the more powerful the beast of bulimia becomes, until its power is so dominant that you must compromise with it and of course, your own obesity.

And still, bulimia can be treated. It takes brains, not brawn, and in order to defeat it you need to get to know it. To recognise its weaknesses, learn how to tame it, find its vulnerable sports, and make plans for its treatment in a "hand to hand" battle with your body. The solutions can be found in you. The secret of winning is to learn to recognise which mechanisms bulimia itself plays on to distract your defences. The first step to success is to reinstate the normal, organic defence mechanisms of your body. Knowledge is power. By acquiring the knowledge, you will gradually manage to outflank your rival and eventually beat it. But always keep in mind that this is a compelling opponent that you will never be able to completely eliminate, but merely tame. However, you must pay attention! An old saying goes, "never make a worthy opponent despair", and we'll come to this later. So, let's start collecting the keys to help us tame bulimia.

3.1.5 Then Let's Just Look at How Glucose and Serotonin Work Together against Bulimia

Let's start right from the moment we sit down at the table and are ready to have a full meal. That is, a meal that combines all three essential food groups with protein, starch, and vitamin C. e.g., chicken with rice and salad. How exactly is a full meal? Let's leave the question come with us further down the line hoping that it will be answered.

Eating food causes blood glucose production. At the same time, the pancreas produces a hormone, insulin, capable of transporting glucose from the blood to the cells and converting it into energy. This mechanism works entirely in the blood (Figure 3.7).

At the same time, another mechanism functions, this time in the brain. Insulin is produced in the pancreas with the help of three other nutrients (Figure 3.8).

1. Amino acids (found in purely protein foods or in combination between cereals or legumes and dairy products),
2. Vitamin C is used as a catalyst (abundant in vegetables, fruits, and fresh juices) and
3. Vitamins of the B complex and in particular Vitamin B6 (pyridoxine) (found in whole grains, raw nuts) all together they produce serotonin in the brain, which is responsible for two critical states: One is the peace of mind and balance in the body, and the other the feeling of satiety.

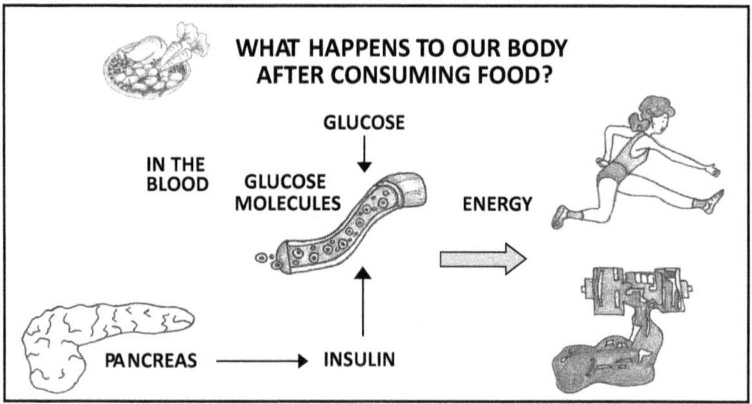

Figure 3.7

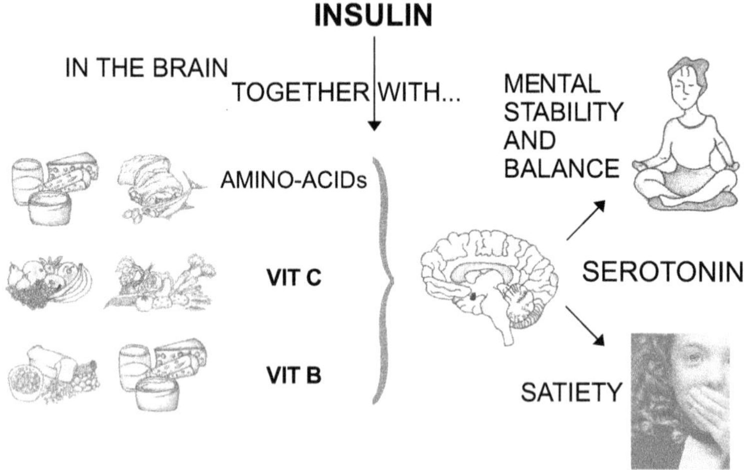

Figure 3.8

The aforementioned serotonin production system is disrupted in people who have made many attempts to lose weight, gone on long-term diets, and mainly unorthodox ones. It takes more than two months of proper nutrition to get the hunger and saturation system back to normal. Failure to adhere to adequate nutrition and the right combination of foods in every meal adds time to the restoration of this mechanism. Thus, it is said that for each day of deviation from proper nutrition and the right combinations of food, one more week is added to the system's recovery, e.g., detoxification diets or chemical diets.

3.1.6 How Much Serotonin Is Enough?

Let's assume that having our full meal (i.e., eating a regular serving of food) provides us with a sufficient serotonin intake, resulting in the brain being given the signal for the two conditions mentioned above (Peace of Mind, Balance and a feeling of Fullness and Satiety) (Figure 3.9).

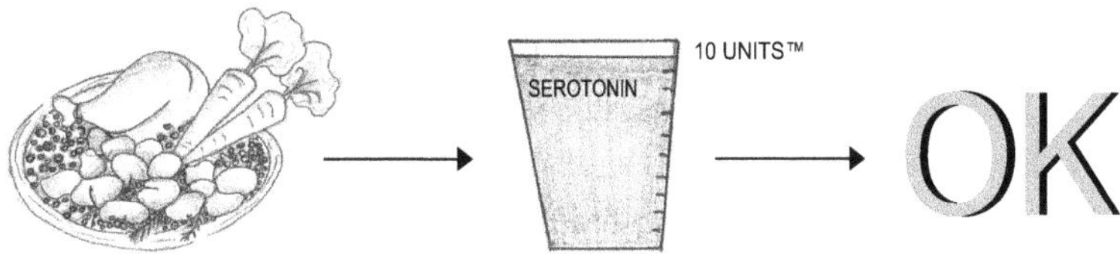

Figure 3.9

Let us now suppose that food consumption is less than average either because of diet or inadequate meals. Then the production of serotonin appears reduced. Suppose it reaches less than 2/3 of the required amount. This leads to unpleasant symptoms such as irritability, insomnia, anxiety (Figure 3.10).

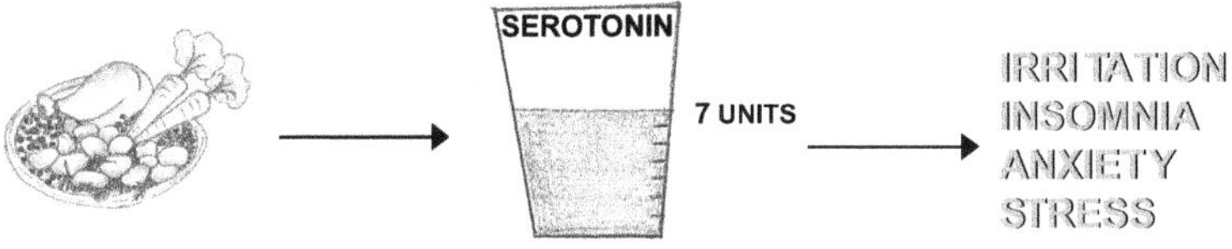

Figure 3.10

In the opposite occasion, when one has consumed twice as much food, there is increased serotonin production as a consequence, and again we have a disorder that is characterized by drowsiness, bad mood and depression. Simultaneously, excess blood glucose due to over-consumption of food that insulin cannot transfer to the cells to produce energy is transported and stored in fat cells (Figure 3.11).

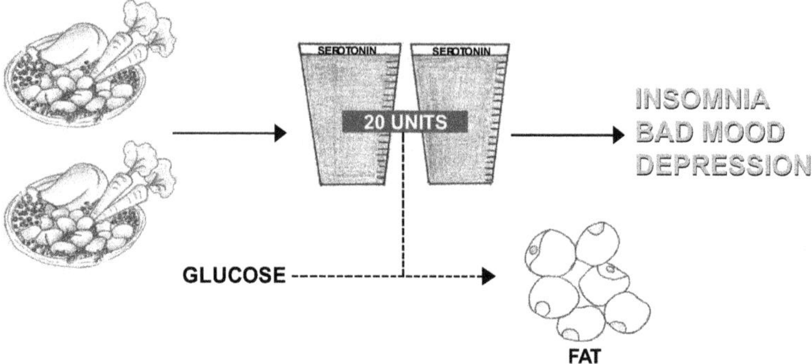

Figure 3.11

It is very frequent for people who have been following a hypocaloric diet for a long time, to find themselves in the intermediate state of reduced serotonin supply to the brain and to experience irritability and stress. For this reason, the goal is for the individual to maintain a permanent production of serotonin, which will, at the same time, ensure the proper function of this mechanism. At the same time, this will also help him lose unnecessary weight without causing further disorder. The role of exercise is vital here. It is preferable to achieve a negative energy equilibrium, mainly due to increased physical activity, rather than dramatically reducing our food intake. That is why all protein diets, monophagia diets and meal replacement diets contribute to the complete disruption of this mechanism, meaning that "the stomach is full, but the mind is hungry".

Both vegetarians and people who frequently have junk food meals can easily fall in this trap of the effects of inadequate meals on mood.

Therefore, this system's function is largely dependent on breakfast. Studies have shown that optimal production and secretion of serotonin is ensured when 30% of the required nutrients of a daily diet are ingested at breakfast. To give a simplified picture of the appropriate and necessary combinations to be followed in the various meals we divided the foods into three major categories (Figure 3.12).

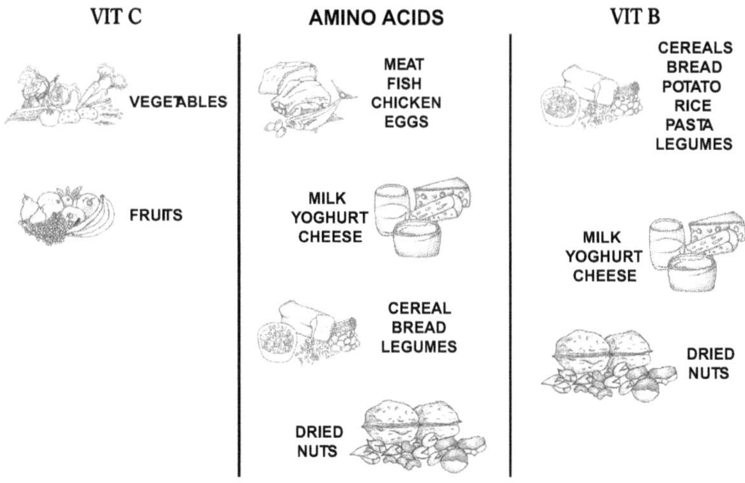

Figure 3.12

3.1.7 The Meal Triads (Groups of Three Types of Food)

This should be included in the so-called "Breakfast Triad" which includes a serving of fruit or fresh juice to provide Vitamin C, a serving of whole grains (bread, nut, toast, breakfast cereals, raw nuts) for half of the essential amino acids but also for the B vitamins and finally a serving of dairy (milk, yoghurt, cheese) for the rest of the amino acids so that we all get all the "essential" amino acids. And all this without taking into account the benefits of other nutrients contained in specific foods such as calcium, protein, fibre, etc.

However, in addition to the "Breakfast Triad", attention should also be paid to the "Meal Triads" (Figure 3.13). For example, for the main meal e.g., lunch, a serving of raw or boiled vegetables, a serving of starchy food (bread, pasta, rice, potato, etc.) and a serving that includes high protein foods such as meat, egg, fish, cheese or a combination of cheese and pulses are required.

For the third meal of the day, that is, the evening or the reversed lunch, it is enough to create a combination like that of breakfast or lunch. We will see some examples of these combinations later.

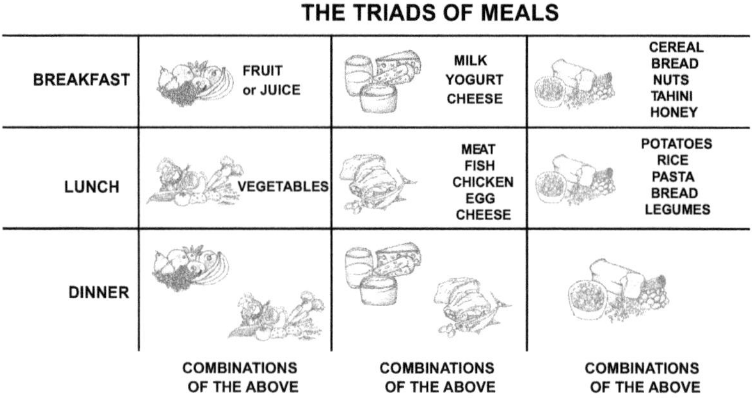

THE TRIADS OF MEALS

BREAKFAST	FRUIT or JUICE	MILK YOGURT CHEESE	CEREAL BREAD NUTS TAHINI HONEY
LUNCH	VEGETABLES	MEAT FISH CHICKEN EGG CHEESE	POTATOES RICE PASTA BREAD LEGUMES
DINNER			
	COMBINATIONS OF THE ABOVE	COMBINATIONS OF THE ABOVE	COMBINATIONS OF THE ABOVE

Figure 3.13

Also, in the time between meals (morning and afternoon) we need to provide a precursor pathway for rapid serotonin production before it is time for lunch or dinner. These snacks between the meals should include at least one fruit or a glass of juice and a small snack rich in complex carbohydrates e.g., a cereal bar, or a small handful of uncooked nuts or a small piece of pasteli or a bun or two spinach or carrot or corn buns or crackers or two digestive biscuits etc., to continuously ensure high levels of serotonin and glucose. If you don't plan the snack, you will not have it. You should always have something with you for emergency cases. Just like when you keep a hidden bill in your wallet. It is also important to know that producing good serotonin takes about 20 minutes to start, which means we have to dedicate time to the meal we have. So, we allow our body to recognize (as in the animal kingdom) the exact amount of food it needs by itself.

By observing the Triads, both in breakfast and in meals, we help the serotonin production system function properly. The hunger and satiety mechanism returns to its normal function providing the body with a multitude of beneficial effects such as wellness and balance and good mood. Let's remember that the traditional Greek diet is so wisely designed with respective combinations such as eating tomatoes (vegetable) with potatoes (starch and half essential amino acids) and cheese (protein and other half amino acids) or eating grilled meat (protein and amino acids) with barley (starch, amino acids) and combine with a seasonal salad (vegetable), etc.

Note: To understand how vital serotonin is, let's just say that it is included in some of the most expensive medicines for treating mental illnesses, the most well-known of which are Ladoz and Prozac, which are mainly serotonergic medicine. Of course, we would not urge anyone to take medication to control their hunger. These medicines are aimed to improve more profound mental disorders. After all, as Hippocrates used to say, "your food is your medicine", and especially regarding serotonin, one would say that he came up with this saying precisely for this mechanism.

The role of chromium in the operation of the aforementioned system is also significant. Chrome is quickly depleted by the increased consumption of simple carbohydrates and mainly sweets, white flour pastries, and soft drinks. But chromium "paves the way" for insulin, which is linked to the transfer and function of glucose to cells and energy production. Unlike chromium, unused glucose is converted into fat stored in the abdomen, hips, buttocks, and thighs. The most crucial chrome food sources are apples, green and red beans, nuts, bananas, broccoli, orange juice, and dietary supplements such as brewer's yeast, spirulina, Zell oxygen, sea-buckthorn, chromium picolinate as a dietary supplement, and others. Nutritional supplements, such as those mentioned above, are characterized by the world bibliography as super foods due to their high nutrient content and particular characteristics as they come from purely natural sources.

Also, cinnamon supplements in tablets have often proved to be particularly beneficial as cinnamon works as a "simulation" of insulin, thereby helping in the best utilization of carbohydrates and significantly reducing hunger, especially during the afternoon. It may not be a coincidence that fatty foods such as stew contain ingredients in their recipe and traditional sweets such as rice pudding, maize cream or traditional halva sprinkled with a little cinnamon.

Before moving on to the dietary pattern, I want to present the amazing properties of certain special foods. Very often, there is a perception that some foods e.g., nuts are fattening. Here we should make the following distinction: Two to three tablespoons of a mixture of raw unsalted nuts may contain the same calories as a cheese pie or a sweet made of white flour and sugar. The difference is that nuts contain the same calories but also a vast range of nutrients such as vitamins, minerals, amino acids, good fats, fibre, which will force the body to utilize all these nutrients immediately. The result will be for the body to put these calories to use during their processing. On the other hand, the cheese pie or sweet cake, containing almost nothing essential and useful for the body, will be turned directly into fat.

This is often the biggest mistake most people make with various diets. For example, they think: "I will not eat what I know is useful, in order to eat what is sweet so I don't get more calories". It's really a tragic mistake. Much preferable and clearly the right way to think is: "I will first eat what is good and nutritious and then whatever more I want". So, keeping your body well-nourished will make you healthier and you will rarely be seduced by eating uncontrolled amounts. Usually when you are given a diet, the standard rule is to follow it and not deviate even in the slightest. While trying to restore hunger and satiety mechanisms with this diet, even if you are on a diet, what you need to do is follow your diet plan carefully and then eat something extra. What ultimately needs to be understood is that the calories that a food or a meal may contain are not so important as their nutrient content. The more the nutrients, the faster the body gains the ability to stop the quantity. Let's think about this a little bit.

3.2 The Smart Food

3.2.1 Are We What We Eat?

This is a question that is answered by another question ... "Do we become what we eat?" If we answer the second question, then we will be led to the solution of the first. So, let's start with the assumption, "What we eat today becomes part of ourselves tomorrow." Let's give some examples to better understand it.

If we consume **calcium**-containing foods today, these foods' calcium will become a new small piece in our bones and teeth.

If we consume fresh fruit today, **Vitamin C** will become an ally in the body's fight against various infections.

If we consume enough **protein** today, then the next day, the damaged tissues will be fully restored, and if we consume more than we need, we will wake up with more stored fat in our body.

If we add two to three tablespoons of raw **olive oil** to our food, our hearts will work better, and our minds will work faster.

If we have **wholegrain foods** daily in our diet, the **B vitamins** will help the body be more active, and our nervous system will be in full clarity and readiness.

If everything we eat today is fresh, without additives and preservatives, it will have positive effects on our mood, our endurance, our mental well-being, and our physical condition. So, I don't know if there is an answer to 'we are what we eat' but indeed what we eat is part of our body and our image.

During the writing of this book, an excellent colleague texted me and came to complete and confirm my thoughts on "The Pharmacy of God." I don't know the author, but it really impressed me, and I would like to share it with you.

3.2.2 God's Pharmacy

A **carrot** slice is like the human eye because it is like watching the apple, the iris, and the pupil!

Science confirms that carrots promote blood flow to the eye and enhance its function.

The **tomato** is red and has four cavities or vents. The heart is also red and has four ventricles. Scientific research shows that tomatoes are an excellent food for the heart and blood.

Grapes form a heart-shaped bunch. Each grape resembles a blood cell and has been proven to be a great food to support and enhance heart function, which also enriches and strengthens the blood.

Walnuts look like a tiny brain with two hemispheres and a cerebellum. Even the walnut's folds give it the look of a brain shell. We know that nuts support the development of neurotransmitters in the brain.

Common **beans** are very similar to human kidneys and actually support their function significantly.

Celery and **rhubarb** look like bones. These foods contribute to the development of strong bones as indicated by their shape.

Eggplants, **avocados**, and **pears** enhance the health and function of the uterus and the cervix. Interestingly, their shape is very reminiscent of this female organ. Today, scientific research has shown that eating an avocado a week helps balance a woman's hormones and helps her lose weight after giving birth and protecting her from cervical cancer. Of particular interest is that avocado blossoms need exactly "9 months" to grow into ripe fruit.

Figs are full of seeds and grow in pairs. Figs boost female fertility, increase sperm motility and thus help fight male infertility.

Olives enhance the health and function of the ovaries.

Grapefruit, **oranges**, and other **citrus fruit** have a striking resemblance to women's mammary glands. They help keep women's breasts healthy and facilitate lymph flow through the breasts' lymphatic system.

Onions are cell shaped. Scientific research has shown that onions help cells get rid of toxins. Also, when we cut them, they produce tears, cleaning the epithelial cells of the eye.

3.2.3 Other Special Foods that Contribute to Combating Eating Disorders in Their Own Way

3.2.3.1 Honey

Honey is one of the most essential products of Greek nature. Although it is similar to sugar, it is not chemically processed and therefore retains all its nutrients. It is an instant source of energy, it has antiseptic properties, antimicrobial activity, and relieves constipation. The minerals it contains are involved in various metabolic processes in the body and regulate stomach acidity.

3.2.3.2 Tahini

Tahini is produced from sesame seed pulp and is the main component of one type of Greek sweet called halva. Tahini contains significant amounts of omega-6 fatty acids, which reduce the levels of 'bad' cholesterol in the blood, responsible for the formation of atherosclerotic plaques. Combined with sesame, a substance with the amazing ability to limit the body's synthesis and absorption, tahini is the perfect food for people seeking to lower cholesterol levels. Tahini is still an essential source of protein (20% content) and vitamins. The vitamin E it contains acts as a powerful antioxidant and helps prevent thrombosis, a property that is further enhanced by lignans of tahini. It contains significant amounts of thiamine (essential for the proper functioning of the nervous system), iron (contributes to optimal physical and mental energy), phosphorus, and calcium (essential for healthy bones and teeth). Tahini can be purchased from any supermarket and organic store. Also remember that traditional pasteli, made exclusively of sesame and honey, can be a great snack in between meals. Also, pasteli made from a mixture of various nuts and sesame has a great nutritional effect as a snack. On the website www.apipharm.gr you will find unique combinations of similar products.

3.2.3.3 Walnut

Walnut is a rich source of omega-6 fatty acids, which reportedly lower "bad" cholesterol levels. It is also a high-protein food (24%) and contains phosphorus and magnesium, essential for good bone health.

3.2.3.4 Almond

Almonds are an excellent source of monounsaturated fatty acids, protein and vitamin E. Indeed, the almond content in vitamin E exceeds even that of olive oil. Almonds also contain lots of vitamins and minerals. Its calcium content covers 25% of the recommended daily intake of 100g. A tablespoon of almonds can be a great snack. It is a good idea to soak them in water for more than an hour to make them more digestible and incredibly nutritious. The water they absorb increases their volume in the stomach, resulting in a prompt feeling of satiety.

3.2.3.5 Hazelnut

Hazelnut contains substantial amounts of Vitamin E, Vitamin B6, folic acid, iron and magnesium. In fact, the vitamin E provided is essential for children as it helps in the proper functioning of the immune system that is developed throughout childhood.

3.2.3.6 Carob syrup

The Carob is a tree that thrives mainly in the Mediterranean, and it seems to become popular in times of war and famine, when food is scarce and difficult to find. This indicates its high nutritional value. Carob syrup also managed to feed John the Baptist in the wilderness and thousands of children during World War II. This is because the flesh of its fruit contains 80% protein, calcium, phosphorus, iron and vitamins. Carob syrup is made by boiling the carob beans and extracting the honey-like substance inside them, whose taste resembles chocolate. But carob syrup is more nutritious than chocolate because it contains 52 times less fat, no oxalic acids, no allergens and caffeine, and its sweetness is owed to natural sugars. Carob syrup is a rich source of carbohydrates, calcium, iron, magnesium, potassium, riboflavin, and low sodium content. Carob flour is also made from carob beans, a flour that can be used to make bread, cakes, biscuits, etc. and gives it a very sweet taste. Carob syrup, like carob flour, can be found in organic stores.

3.2.3.7 Flaxseed

Flaxseed is food with valuable nutrients and proven beneficial effects on human health. More than 50% of flaxseed consists of omega-3 fatty acids that significantly reduce "bad" cholesterol. It also contains omega-6 and monounsaturated fatty acids. Flaxseed is also the primary source of lignans, substances with potent antioxidant properties that appear to have beneficial effects against breast cancer development and other types of cancer. It is low in sodium and does not contain gluten, making flour more digestible and especially suitable for people with gluten intolerance. Flaxseed also contains 27% dietary fibre, which is essential for the proper function of the digestive system. Lastly, flaxseed is a protein-rich food (includes 18% protein) that contains all the essential amino acids in sufficient quantities. Since it is difficult to be absorbed in its natural form, you need to grind it into dust in a blender or coffee grinder and then either mix it with other ground nuts or add it to salads or cook with food ingredients, such as legumes, enhancing the nutritional value of your meals. Usually, half a teaspoon per meal is a sufficient amount to receive the beneficial effect of its ingredients. You can find it in all organic stores.

3.2.3.8 Flaxseed oil

Flaxseed oil, that is, oil from flaxseed grinding, contains some phytoestrogens that either prevent cancer or slow its progression, lower cholesterol levels, and boost the immune system. As colleague Vasiliki Karasmanoglou characteristically mentions in the 20th issue of the journal Diatrofi. Health & Wellness", according to studies presented at the conference of the American Society for Cancer Research, omega-3, fatty acids may protect women from breast cancer. Additionally, flaxseed oil is rich in calcium, vitamin E and protein. Recent research has reached positive results regarding its therapeutic effects on psychiatric and neurological problems, such as depression and bipolar disorder.

Flaxseed oil helps:

- to treat constipation
- in the treatment of irritable bowel syndrome
- in the treatment of asthma
- the heart
- the immune system (studies have shown that children who ate a teaspoon of yogurt with linseed oil every morning had less and milder respiratory problems during the school year)
- with menstrual pain
- the skin, in cases of eczema and dry skin
- against heart disease
- cut the craving for unhealthy fats
- to balance blood sugar
- against hypertension
- increase the body's metabolism
- burn unhealthy fats in the body
- thermogenesis
- against high cholesterol or triglycerides

Finally, it has been shown to aid in treating prostate cancer and acting against HIV / AIDS. An ideal way to consume it is for each raw spoonful of olive oil that you add to your meal you add one teaspoon of linseed oil. You will find it mainly in organic stores.

3.2.3.9 Olive oil

Olive oil, a major ingredient of the Mediterranean Diet, is the richest source of monounsaturated fatty acids, which reduce "bad" cholesterol and triglyceride levels while maintaining "good" cholesterol levels. Olive oil is rich in all fat-soluble vitamins and especially in antioxidant vitamin E. It has been shown that olive oil increases the body's resistance helps the central nervous system function correctly and reduces heart problems.

3.2.3.10 Cocoa

Cocoa contains significant amounts of iron, magnesium, phosphorus and potassium. A hot drink with two teaspoons of cocoa, a teaspoon of black sugar and some milk, fresh or condensed, in the afternoon can stimulate the body, but also prevent craving for chocolate. It can also superbly replace afternoon coffee without adversely affecting sleep quality, as the caffeine it contains can invigorate the body without adversely affecting the nervous system.

3.2.3.11 Chocolate, the misunderstood

Chocolate is one of the most misunderstood foods. As you will see below, consuming a small amount daily can have very beneficial effects. As colleague, Christina Dranitsa, mentions in the 4th issue of Diatrofi. Health & Wellness", we have selected the most exciting information for you, so that you know how much and to what effect you can consume it safely. Chocolate is made from seeds of the tropical cocoa tree, whose scientific name is Theobroma cacao. The word Theobroma cacao is of Greek origin. It comes from the words "god" and consumption ("vrosi" in Greek) and means food for the gods. Chocolate was introduced to Europe in the 16th century by marine researchers, where it quickly became widely known. Today it is the most popular food for women and the second most popular for men.

It contains proteins, carbohydrates and fats and is a rich source of energy. In addition to the aforementioned calorie-rich ingredients, chocolate also contains vitamins [A, D and E, B-complex vitamins (thiamine, riboflavin, etc.), minerals and trace elements (potassium, sodium, calcium, magnesium, iron, copper, zinc). Chocolate also contains theobromine (a substance that stimulates the nervous system and the kidneys, acting as a light diuretic) as well as polyphenols (substances that are known for their antioxidant properties and are thought to inhibit the activity of oral bacteria).

Chocolate, as mentioned above, is a rich source of nutrients. But what are its elements that lead us to desire it so much? It is believed to contain over 300 substances that act on the human central nervous system. For example, it contains tryptophan, an amino acid converted into serotonin in the body (a substance that causes us to feel exulted and ecstatic and is considered a key to treating depression). Chocolate is also a natural source of phenylethylamine, a substance that is believed to have psychostimulant properties. In addition to the aforementioned substances, chocolate also contains other substances that act on our brains, resulting in the release of endorphins (natural hormones of our body analogous to morphine and making us happy).

3.2.3.12 Myths and Facts

- There is no direct evidence that chocolate causes tooth problems.
- Chocolate has been accused of causing headaches and migraines. Scientifically, this has not been substantiated.
- Chocolate allergy is one of the rarest forms of allergy. Usually, the milk and nuts chocolate products often contain are the leading causes of such reactions.
- Finally, a belief that has dominated people's opinions for several decades is that chocolate causes acne. Scientific research has also disproven this myth. Summing up, we conclude that chocolate is one of the most misunderstood foods. While it is accused of causing many problems, it is "almost" harmless. But, like all foods, it should always be consumed in moderation. An amount of 10-15 grams three to four times a week is ideal.

3.2.3.13 Tea: More than a simple beverage

Tea, as described by colleagues Katerina Karakike and Katerina Hadou in the 11th issue of the journal Diatrofi. Health & Wellness", begins its journey in history one day in 2737 BC, when the leaves of a tropical tree, ubiquitous in southwestern China, were dragged and dropped into the cup of boiling water by the Emperor Shen Nung. Immediately a delicate scent emerged, and the water had an excellent and mild taste.

Tea is produced from the leaves of a single species of tree, the Camellia Sinensis. Despite this, however, two tea types are never the same, even though they come from the same area and the same plantation. Its quality, aroma, and taste vary greatly depending on the country of origin and the type of leaf. The fermentation process is responsible for the different kinds of tea: White, black, green, oolong.

- White tea is made from young plant buds that have not been oxidized. It is produced in much smaller quantities than other types and is therefore much more expensive and less widespread.
- Green tea is made from leaves that have been slightly oxidized.
- Black tea, whose leaves have been heavily oxidized under controlled temperature and humidity conditions, which cause enzymatic reactions, resulting in alteration of the colour of the leaf.
- Colonial tea, which is the result of the oxidation process being interrupted between green and black tea. Tea is not only known for its aroma and taste but also for its beneficial properties.

It contains significant amounts of a class of polyphenols called flavonoids. More and more scientific studies prove the significant antioxidant activity of flavonoids.

Tea consumption has been associated with strengthening our immune system, protecting our teeth from plaque and gingivitis but also reducing the risk of cardiovascular disease. At the same time, experimental data confirm vasoconstrictive, anti-thrombotic and anti-inflammatory inflammation. It seems that consuming 3 cups of tea a day can reduce the risk of heart attack by 11%.

Drinking tea can help the body get **hydrated**. Many studies have shown that moderate tea consumption of 4 to 6 cups helps maintain body fluid homoeostasis. Also, any herbal infusion with traditional herbs such as mountain tea and sage or a blend of them in the morning, or chamomile in the evening is a wonderful choice consumed without sweeteners or with a little honey or black sugar.

A warm chamomile infusion with a teaspoon of honey before bed is a beautiful soothing for the nervous and digestive system.

A great idea is to combine our meals with an infusion because we can improve digestion and avoid the consumption of alcohol. Another good idea is to prepare a large quantity and place it in glass bottles in the fridge; this way, we can either warm up the serving we want to drink or consume it as cold or iced tea.

A good recipe is to boil 3 litres of water for two to three minutes adding ten mountain tea sticks. After removing it from the hotplate, add two or three sachets of green tea or green tea with catechin. Infuse it for a maximum of 3 minutes to avoid bitterness but leave the mountain tea in the hot water. After waiting for at least an hour for the infusion to cool, add three tablespoons of honey. Allow it to cool for at least another two hours, strain it, and store it in glass bottles in the refrigerator.

Another great idea is to put a few sticks of mountain tea and/ or other herbs in the glass jug of a coffee maker and just activate the device. Without removing the herbs from the water and leaving the coffee maker on, you will have ready-made tea you can drink unsweetened or with little honey. The infusion that results from the prolonged refining of the herbs in hot water is truly a fantastic tasting experience.

It may not be a coincidence that most people in eastern countries use it in every meal, in areas where obesity rates are minimal. For example, although living in one of the most developed countries in the world, the Japanese have the lowest obesity and highest longevity rates world-wide, as their diet is based primarily on eating fish, fruits and vegetables. One feature is that they consume an average of two cups of tea per hour. In fact, for this habit, a company made a teapot which they called i-pot to protect the elderly. The device sends a distress signal online to the closest relatives of the elderly person when they find that they have spent enough time without drinking their traditional tea.

Tea is more than just a beverage with beneficial health effects: it is the inspiration for a better and calmer lifestyle.

3.2.4 Milk Fermentation Products (Yoghurt, Sour Milk, Ayran, Kefir)

Yoghurt, sour milk, Ayran and **kefir** are fermented milk yeast products. They are milk derivatives when fermented using appropriate fermentation of microorganisms. Any milk fermentation product can be assumed to have the same nutritional value as milk. However, the fermentation of microorganisms causes significant changes in the composition of milk. Yogurt, which is the most well-known variant of these foods (not being superior to any of the others) is excellent food with multiple health benefits.

- Yoghurt proteins are of superior biological value to the milk proteins of which it is made. They are digested in half the time and are used more quickly by the body.
- Yoghurt can also be consumed by people who suffer from lactose intolerance without unpleasant symptoms (abdominal pain, cramps, diarrhoea).
- The increased presence of lactic acid in yoghurt and other fermented milk products results in better absorption of calcium, iron and phosphorus in the food.
- The lactic acid found in yoghurt and other fermented milk products also causes a higher production of gastric juices, resulting in faster digestion.

Milk fermentation products also:

- Help in the treatment of gastrointestinal disorders (poisoning, diarrhoea, constipation).
- Have antibiotic effect in the gut area.
- Probably lower cholesterol.
- Have anti-cancer properties.
- Renew and restore the gut microbial flora The microorganisms present in the gastrointestinal tract have many beneficial effects on the human body.
- Help in regular and smooth bowel movement. The possible mechanism is that their action helps in increasing the volume of intestinal contents and thus create more stimulation.
- The content of the gastrointestinal tract, with the influence of microorganisms, becomes softer. This results in less irritation when passing through the intestine.
- They prevent the development of pathogenic microorganisms that cause diarrhoea.
- They retain water, thereby reducing its amount in the intestinal tract, thereby reducing the likelihood for diarrhoea.

Kefir as described by colleague Aphrodite Iliadou in the 18th issue of the journal "Diatrofi. Health & Wellness", like all milk fermentation products, is a natural dairy product that the indigenous people of the

Caucasus and the Middle East have been consuming and enjoying for many centuries now. It is also common for residents of these areas to be over 100 years old.

Although milk is an excellent food, the fermentation of kefir grains actually "upgrades" it. Kefir seeds are a mass of bacteria, yeast and polysaccharide and their microbiology is very complex. The polysaccharide in the kefir seed mass is unique and has been given the name "Kerifan".

The particularity of kefir is that it is easily digested by the body - more than yogurt, cleanses the intestines, provides beneficial bacteria, yeasts, vitamins, minerals and high-value proteins. It is a fully balanced source of nutrition and contributes to a healthy immune system. It is said that regular use of kefir can help relieve all intestinal disorders, promote bowel movement, create a healthy digestive system free from constipation. It is one of the best probiotic and antioxidant foods, it affects the whole body and helps maintain a balanced inner ecosystem for optimal health and longevity. Highly recommended for infants, pregnant women and the elderly. Its beneficial yeasts and friendly bacteria consume most of the lactose of milk. Thus, it is ideal for people who are lactose intolerant.

It provides plenty of calcium, magnesium, phosphorus for proper cell growth, body maintenance, and abundant energy. Kefir is rich in vitamin B12, B1, and an excellent source of biotin that helps the body absorb other B vitamins.

According to all research, kefir has many beneficial properties such as:

- It improves conditions like anaemia.
- It helps with digestive tract diseases, chronic enteritis, kidney and liver diseases.
- It has diuretic properties.
- It helps the recovery from various illnesses and generally benefits the human body.
- It is an excellent food very low in fat and calories.
- It is an ideal product with a high nutritional value for those involved in sports.
- Frequent use helps to fight atherosclerosis and hypertension.
- It helps restore the inner ecosystem after antibiotic therapy.

Other potential benefits that have also been reported are its cancer-preventing effect, and lowering of blood cholesterol levels, which are said to treat and heal rashes and eczema by placing kefir on the affected area. You can buy kefir seeds from organic stores and grow it yourself at home or get the ready-made kefir beverage on the market.

3.2.5 Methuselah's Lunch (One Image, a Thousand Nutrients)

Methuselah became known in history as one of the longest living humans on earth. In the book of Genesis, he is mentioned as the son of Enoch and the father of Lamech, whom he had at the age of 187. Bible scholars argue that he died shortly before the onset of the Flood.

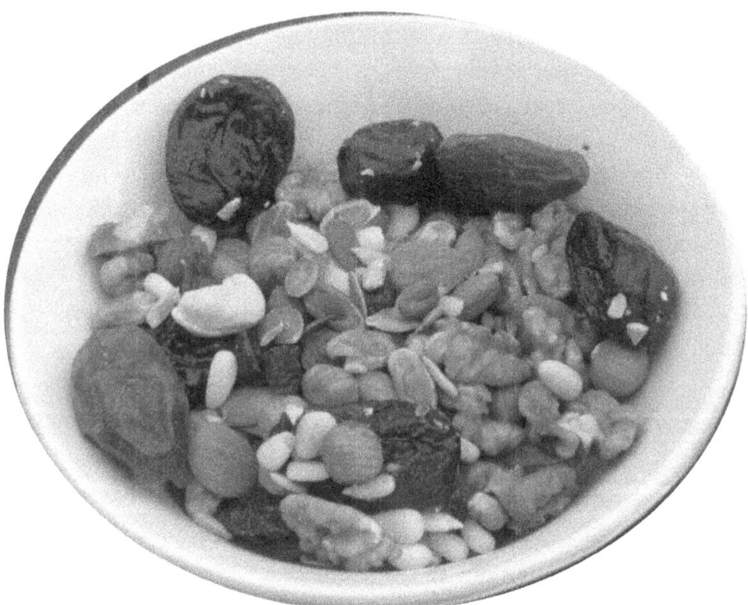

Figure 3.14

Regardless of wanting to surpass Methuselah or not, on would undoubtedly be interested in having Methuselah's performance. One of the most appropriate ways to achieve this is to include in his daily diet a small bowl of unsalted nuts and dried fruit. The picture shown in Figure 3.14 speaks for itself. Empty several bags of walnuts, almonds, caseous, macadamia walnuts, hazelnuts, sunflower seeds, pumpkin seed, pine nuts, pistachios, dried plums, raisins, dates, cranberries, etc. into a large container and every morning before leaving for work, school or during your afternoon errands, fill your pocket with about half the size of a 200g yoghurt carton and supply your body with a variety of vitamins, minerals, amino acids, good fatty acids and energy that will make you stand out for your performance. These nuts can stimulate the production of acetylcholine. This substance helps increase concentration, improve memory, increase endurance, and promote good mood. This small meal would be more beneficial if you consumed it for a period of one to two hours and not within ten minutes to get a long extension of your strength. This extended meal will also help you eliminate the bulimia crises that occur when we return home after several hours of staying on an empty stomach for a long time.

3.3 Key Takeaways

1. **Your relationship with food can change:**
    - Learn to trust in your body's natural ability to regulate hunger and fullness.
    - When you focus on your body's needs instead of external influences, you build a healthier connection with food.
2. **Listen to your body:**
    - Instead of following strict diets, pay attention to the signals your body gives you, like hunger and satisfaction after meals.
    - Natural, wholesome foods are your best allies in finding this balance.
3. **Small changes, big results:**
    - Start with small, simple adjustments to your diet that make you feel good. They will, in time, lead to bigger ones
    - Remember, every step you take toward a more nourishing diet is a win.

4. **Food is more than fuel; it's a companion:**
    - See food as a means of not only physical but also emotional nourishment.
    - Enjoy the process of choosing, preparing, and eating food without guilt.
5. **Give yourself time:**
    - Change doesn't happen overnight. Whether you're trying to repair your relationship with food or improve your diet, allow yourself to progress at your own pace.
6. **Don't hesitate to seek support:**
    - The journey to better nutrition doesn't have to be a solo one. Professionals can guide and support you along the way.

Chapter 4

Diet Model for the Treatment of Eating Disorders

It is not enough to properly nourish only the body, but the mind and soul as well.

4.1 Sample Diet

As soon as you wake up, drink a glass of water, and then you can then make a selection from each column.

Before each meal you should always drink a glass of water

- A prerequisite for uplifting your body in combination with the proper nutrition, as suggested further in the book, is sufficient rest that will be ensured with a minimum of 6 hours of continuous night sleep.
- On a day you follow a 60-minute exercise plan, eat a fruit or drink a small carton of juice immediately after exercising.
- During exercise, if it lasts more than 60 minutes, drink a 500-1000 ml mix of 50% water & 50% juice instead of 500-1000 ml of plain water.
- Try to accompany all your meals with a cup of unsweetened tea or mixed with half a teaspoon of black sugar or honey.
- All legumes should be soaked in water for two days before they are cooked.

Nutritional Intelligence: The Answer to Bulimia, Overeating, and Obesity
Evangelos Zoumbaneas

ISBN 978-981-5129-74-8 (Hardcover), 978-981-5129-73-1 (Paperback), 978-1-003-65188-8 (eBook)
www.jennystanford.com

BREAKFAST OPTIONS e.g., 8:00-8:30	**Breakfast e.g., 10:00-10:30**	**Meal options e.g., 15:00-15:30**	**AFTERNOON e.g., 17:30-18:00**	**DINNER OPTIONS or replace with lunch options**
A cup of milk with four spoons of cereal a teaspoon of mixed nuts and a fruit.	A fruit **and** a 1st choice snack like a small bowl of mixed nuts and dried fruit	Salad with two spoons of olive oil and two medium sized burgers **and** a slice of bread or a teacup of rice with vegetables or corn	Two fruits **and** a small bowl of mixed nuts and dried fruit, **or** a snack, **or** a glass of juice in the blender (see below).	A salad with mixed vegetables, a serving of cheese, and a slice of bread or a medium sized rusk **or** a tomato salad with five olives, a serving of feta cheese and a slice of bread or a medium sized rusk
Two melba toasts or slices of wholegrain bread with a teaspoon of tahini and honey **or** margarine and a teaspoon of honey and a teaspoon of mixed nuts and a fruit.		Potato salad made with two medium sized potatoes, fresh vegetables with two spoons of olive oil, one egg **and** a serving of cheese.		A Cretan rusk with around 100 grams of cottage cheese or a serving of feta cheese of around 50 grams with half a tomato (grated) and a spoon of olive oil.
Some fruit, a small carton of milk and four digestive biscuits with honey or a pasteli bar (up to 25 grams)	During working days around **12:30-13:00**, an additional fruit and a snack (see below)	Salad with two spoons of olive oil **with** a serving of fish **and** a slice of bread or a teacup of rice with vegetables **or** a medium sized boiled potato.		A tuna salad with fresh vegetables and Alfa Alfa sprouts and a teaspoon of corn. Two grilled chicken or pork skews with one grilled pita and a small salad.
A yogurt with a teaspoon of honey, a digestive biscuit and two teaspoons of mixed, ground dried nuts and a fruit.		Salad with two teaspoons of olive oil **and** a serving of meat **and** a teacup of brown rice or pasta or a medium sized baked potato.		An individual pita or an Arabic pita baked in the oven with slices of tomato, two slices of cheese, one slice of turkey ham, mushrooms, chopped pepper, etc.

BREAKFAST OPTIONS e.g., 8:00-8:30	Breakfast e.g., 10:00-10:30	Meal options e.g., 15:00-15:30	AFTERNOON e.g., 17:30-18:00	DINNER OPTIONS or replace with lunch options
A sandwich with turkey, cheese and a vegetable and a fruit or a fresh juice.	A fresh fruit accompanied by a home-made cereal bar	Two cups of salad with rice or pasta with two spoons of olive oil **and** a serving of cheese **and** an egg or two slices of less fatty turkey cold cut.	Two fresh fruit and a small bowl of mixed nuts and dried fruit, or a snack or a glass of blended fruit juice.	A small bowl of yoghurt with a spoon of cereal and two teaspoons of ground mixed dried nuts, a teaspoon of honey and some fruit.
A bowl of quacker with a fruit and a teaspoon of honey and a teaspoon of ground mixed dried nuts.	Between 12:30-13:00 another fresh fruit with a handful of dried nuts	Salad with two spoons of olive oil **and** a serving of chicken **and** one medium sized baked potato or a teacup of potato puree or peas or rice with mixed vegetables.		A boiled or poached egg on a slice of bread vegetables. (On a day that you don't have meat or fish).
Two large crispy bread sticks with sunflower seed or a medium sized rusk and a serving of cheese and a fruit or fresh juice.		A salad with two spoons of olive oil with fresh vegetables and Alfa Alfa sprouts **with** a teaspoon of boiled legumes and a serving of chicken or tuna or salmon.		An omelette with vegetables with a serving of cheese **and** a slice of bread (On a day that you don't have meat or fish).

BREAKFAST OPTIONS **e.g., 8:00-8:30**	**Breakfast** **e.g., 10:00-10:30**	**Meal options** **e.g., 15:00-15:30**	**AFTERNOON** **e.g., 17:30-18:00**	**DINNER OPTIONS** **or replace with lunch options**
A small bowl of yoghurt or rice pudding and a crispy bread stick or a digestive biscuit or a wholegrain biscuit and a fruit.	A fresh fruit accompanied by a home-made cereal bar	Two cups of peas with potato and carrot or two cups of fresh peas and a small sized potato **or** two cups of Imam **or** two medium sized stuffed vegetables with a small sized potato with one serving of cheese **and** a slice of bread.	Two fresh fruit and a small bowl of mixed nuts and dried fruit, or a snack or a glass of blended fruit juice.	One of the breakfast options **or** the half of a lunch option.
Two melba toasts or slices of wholegrain bread and a serving of cheese and a fruit or fresh juice.	Between 12:30–13:00 another fresh fruit with a handful of dried nuts	Salad with two spoons of olive oil **with** two cups of boiled pasta **with** three spoons of salsa or minced meat **and** a spoon of grated cheese.		Half of a medium sized avocado with a teaspoon of honey **with** two teaspoons of mixed dried nuts.

BREAKFAST OPTIONS e.g., 8:00-8:30	**Breakfast e.g., 10:00-10:30**	**Meal options e.g., 15:00-15:30**	**AFTERNOON e.g., 17:30-18:00**	**DINNER OPTIONS or replace with lunch options**
Two melba toasts or slices of bread with 30 grams of halva, or two teaspoons of tahini and honey or peanut butter and one fruit.		Two cups of boiled legumes (one cup of lentils, beans or chickpeas and one cup of liquid) **and** a serving of cheese or half a serving of fish **with** five large olives and a thin slice of wholegrain bread.		A serving of vegetable soup or a cup of fava beans **or** black-eyes peas with one rusk **and** five olives.
Two large crispy bread sticks with sunflower seeds or a medium sized rusk with two teaspoons of mixed dried nuts and a fruit or fresh juice.		A small sized serving of calamari cooked in tomato sauce with a cup of rice or orzo **or** two cups of macaroni with octopus or calamari **and** a slice of bread.		Two small sized potatoes with two spoons of olive oil **and** a medium sized tomato **and** five olives.
A cup of cereal with dried nuts and raisins and a fruit or fresh juice.		Two artichokes with potato and carrot or a teacup of spinach with rice with one rusk, a slice of bread and five olives.		

- Place the legumes in a pan and add a cup of water. Whenever they absorb the water, we add a little more. E.g., we start the process on Monday night and cook them on Tuesday night or better on Wednesday. This way, they become more digestible and release more nutrients. (if you want to supplement this meal with a salad it is optional)

During the day, in between meals, you can choose from the following snacks:

- Two tablespoons of a mixture of **almond nuts, sunflower seeds, pumpkin seed, pistachio nuts, cashew nuts, cranberries, raisins, macadamia, pecan, dates, etc. (see Methuselah's secret)**
- or **twenty almonds** thoroughly washed and soaked in some water for at least 30 minutes to make them more digestible and more nutritious
- or a **pasteli** bar (appr. 20g)
- or **two biscuits or a wholegrain biscuit or two wholegrain biscuits that you can both stuff with a teaspoon of honey and nuts**
- or a **small bun**
- or a **wholegrain cereal bar**
- or two **wholegrain crackers**
- or two large **crispy bread sticks** or three small ones
- or a small piece of homemade **apple pie or cake** you can make with whole grain flour.

A prerequisite for the success of your program is: having an extra physical activity e.g., workout or walking, etc. At least for 30 minutes five to six times a week.

If you dine out, you can either adjust the options above or use the following suggestions:

(a) eat a large mixed salad with a serving of roasted meat and up to 10 mouthfuls (forkfuls, bites or whatever you like) or (b) eat up to 20 mouthfuls of whatever you want. If is the meal includes a sweet, you will eat an extra 5 mouthfuls. The salads are meant to be plentiful on the table and are not included in the 10 or 20 mouthfuls. If you have a buffet to choose from, mentally divide your plate in two, fill half of it with the salads and make a small combination in the other half according to the aforementioned suggestions. Then take another plate and repeat the process with different foods. The overfilled plate of mixed foods alters the flavours and forces you to eat more. Alternatively, you could eat two skewers with a grilled pita or a grilled pita with a skewer and a salad if possible.

How to prepare:

a. yogurt with cereal and grated dried nuts
   Add to yoghurt of up to 4% fat content, a blend of Methuselah's secret and allow two to three hours to soak in the yoghurt mix or add two spoonfuls of breakfast cereal, a teaspoon of honey and two teaspoons of ground walnuts, almonds (grind 30 almonds, 5 walnuts, 5 hazelnuts, 1 tablespoon of flaxseed, and store in the refrigerator so that you will use the quantity you need each time). Finish with a small or half a large chopped fruit and you will have an excellent full meal.
b. juice with various fruits (e.g., a banana, an orange, an apple or a pear) and half a serving of yoghurt, add water equal to 1 yogurt container a few ice cubes and a tablespoon of honey. Mix the ingredients for about a minute and prepare 2 servings.

4.2 Quantities and Servings

4.2.1 What Is a "Serving" of Food?

It is imperative to know how much food you need without help. The best way to achieve this is to combine all of the above. That is, having a good breakfast, having plenty of fruit and/or juice snacks and chewing food well will help you get a "personal appetite and satiety regulator" and you'll see that soon you will know how much of the served food you need.

But for some food, such as meat, fish or cheese, it would be good to have a sense of how much of them we need. Since we consider weighing food a "compulsive method," **we will give you a way to calculate the proper servings based on your physique**. For example, if we were to serve a steak to a 1.85 tall man and a 1.60 tall woman clearly and fairly, we would choose a larger one for the former and a smaller one for the latter.

One practical way to calculate servings based on our physique is:

To calculate the s**erving of meat**, we form a circle, bringing our index finger and our thumb together. This circle, which is about as thick as index finger, measures about as much as a medium sized boneless steak. The same volume fits two or three small burgers or a small or large chicken breast, always depending on the size of each person's fingers.

In the same way, we can calculate the amount of a **serving of fish**, we will only use the larger circle formed by the thumb and the middle of the fingers instead of the index finger. Picture this size, as a fish, without a head and tail or a perch or swordfish or salmon fillet. Simply put, because fish has much less fat than meat, we can always eat a little more.

With a different finger formation, we can calculate a **serving of cheese**. If we combine the three fingers: index, middle and ring finger from the base to the top of the fingers, a volume of about a rectangle or even more plainly, a piece of feta cheese that we add, for example, in a Greek salad. Suppose the cheese is hard like Gruyere or Kefalotyri. In that case, we calculate the serving based on the volume formed by the index and middle fingers. And that's because the harder a cheese is, the more fat it contains.

The **size of a potato** where it is mentioned will be calculated similar to a tennis ball by volume.

The **amount of a cup** will refer to the same volume as a single-serving yoghurt container weighing 150-200 g.

All other quantities will refer to teaspoons or tablespoons.

You can find more information, suggestions, ideas and combinations either in the book *Chef... in the Nick of Time"* or in *What Will You Cook Today, Mom* by Metaichmion Publications, or in the official website www.diatrofi.gr

4.2.2 Chapter 4 Outline

This book was written for women suffering from an eating disorder. Not because there are no men who suffer from the same disorders and who clearly need specialists, but women are always the first and most "targeted" victims of what is termed as the "slimming industry". The information and examples described in this book concern both women and men. Under the same biochemical mechanisms, we are all affected precisely the same, with the same effects that inadvertently or voluntarily create imbalances within our bodies. Clearly, all information applies equally to any person who has been bound by an eating disorder, as it does to anyone who would like to avoid getting involved in such unpleasant situations.

In my twenty years of experience as a dietitian, I have seen people losing a lot of weight and after a few years gaining that weight again. This is, unfortunately, the situation of those people who finally managed to achieve the coveted slimming result. The statistics are tragic. Out of the 100 people who start a slimming program, about ten will eventually reach their goal. Out of these ten, statistically, only “one” manages to maintain his weight forever. Conclusion? About one in a hundred people, that is, only 1%, achieve the real goal, to radically change their eating habits and maintain an ideal body weight forever.

Practically, the first information every person who decides to get on a diet plan is interested in is how much weight he will lose and when. But no one ever informs him that going into this process, he is likely to develop some kind of eating disorder because the diet process itself is an abnormal parameter for living being. No one informs the person who is willing to lose weight that during the diet there will also be periods that will negatively affect his mood, there will come days that he will feel tired, nights that he will lose sleep, times when he will lose his temper, he will face situations that will make him lose his temper, he will be forced to spend hours that will feel like hell and finally he will return to his former state, from which he may never come back.

Voluntary starvation does not exist in nature. The wildest animals, when deprived of food, become even more ferocious until they are satiated. Diet itself is a highly wearing condition for both physical and mental health. Therefore, it should take place under the guidance and supervision of specialized therapists who consider all the negative factors that may affect its course. The faster the slimming, the more probable the appearance of an eating disorder is. The slower the process is, combined with physical activity and under the supervision of a qualified nutritionist, the more confidently one will achieve his goal. As for the final result? That is to say, maintaining the ideal weight after the end of a diet forever ... no one can be sure. This is what we will discuss in the next chapter.

4.2.3 From Theory to Practice

The following lists the authentic daily logs of the proper daily application of the suggested diet.

WEEK						
Monday 31/5/2010	**Tuesday 1/6/2010**	**Wednesday 2/6/2010**	**Thursday 3/6/2010**	**Friday 4/6/2010**	**Saturday 5/6/2010**	**Sunday 6/6/2010**
Breakfast	Breakfast	Breakfast	Breakfast	Breakfast	Breakfast	Breakfast
7:00:1 petite beurre cookie + 2 melba toast + 1 slice of bread + little margarine + honey + cup of coffee – milk + half a banana + half an apple.	7:00: 2 melba toast + half a banana + marmalade + 1 cup of milk.	7:00: 2 melba toast + marmalade + 1 cup of milk + half a banana.	7:00: 2 melba toast + marmalade + 1 cup of milk + half a banana.	7:00: 2 melba toast + marmalade + 1 cup of coffee with milk + half a banana + 2 small rusks.	7:00: 2 melba toast + 1 teaspoon of marmalade + 1 cup of coffee + half a banana + 1 digestive cookie.	7:00: 1 melba toast + marmalade + 2 rusks + half a banana + tea.
snack	snack	snack	snack	snack	snack	snack
11:00: Peach juice + 2 petit beurre cookies.	11:00: 1 apple + 1 bun	11:00: 2 apricots + petit beurre cookies.	11:00: 2 apricots + 2 petit beurre cookies.	11:00: 2 apricots + 2 petit beurre cookies.	11:00: 2 apricots + 2 petit beurre cookies.	11:00: 1 peach + 2 melba toast + dried nuts (1 tablespoon).
Meal	Meal	Meal	Meal	Meal	Meal	Meal
15:00: a portion of horse beans + 1 rusk.	15:00: 2 pieces of cheese pie + salad.	14:45: Pork + salad + a potato.	15:00: Boiled chicken (1 portion) + pasta + salad.	15:00: A piece of chicken + salad (no oil) + 1 slice of bread.	15:00: A portion of veal + 1 potato + celery + carrot + ½ glass of beer.	15:00: A portion of veal + 3 tablespoons of orzo + salad.

WEEK						
Monday 31/5/2010	**Tuesday 1/6/2010**	**Wednesday 2/6/2010**	**Thursday 3/6/2010**	**Friday 4/6/2010**	**Saturday 5/6/2010**	**Sunday 6/6/2010**
snack	snack	snack	snack	snack	snack	snack
18:00: 2 apricots + 2 petit beurre cookies.	18:00: 2 apricots + 2 anise rusks.	18:30: 2 apricots + 2 petit beurre cookies.	18:30: 2 apricots + 2 petit beurre cookies.	18:00: 2 melba toast + 1 peach.	18:00: 3 apricots + 2 digestive cookies + 1 cookie with almonds.	18:00: 1 apple + 2 cookies.
dinner	dinner	dinner	dinner	dinner	dinner	dinner
22:00: Yoghurt + 2 melba toast + marmalade (a teaspoon, home-made).	22:30: Yoghurt (2% fat) + 2 melba toast.	22:30: 3 bites of pork + salad + rusk.	22:30: 1/4 portion of chicken + salad + rusk + 1 melba toast + marmalade.	22:00: 3 pieces of thin dough pizza + a glass of beer.	22:00: Vegetables (carrot and celery) + 1 piece of cheese + 1 slice of bread.	22:00: 1 tomato + 1 piece of cheese + 1 slice of bread.
Physical activity	Physical activity	Physical activity	Physical activity	Physical activity	Physical activity	Physical activity
Type: Walking Duration: 45 mins	Type: Walking Duration: 40 mins	Type: - Duration: -	Type: Walking Duration: 15 mins	Type: - Duration: -	Type: - Duration: -	Type: - Duration: -

WEEK						
Monday	**Tuesday**	**Wednesday**	**Thursday**	**Friday**	**Saturday**	**Sunday**
Breakfast	Breakfast	Breakfast	Breakfast	Breakfast	Breakfast	Breakfast
Milk, 2 digestive cookies, 1 nectarine.	Milk, 2 cream crackers, 1 nectarine.	Milk, 2 home-made cookies, 1 nectarine.	Milk, 2 home-made cookies, 1 nectarine.	1 glass of milk, 2 digestive cookies, 1 nectarine.	1 glass of milk, 2 home-made cookies, some grapes.	1 glass of milk, 1 slice of bread with honey, 1 nectarine
snack	snack	snack	snack	snack	snack	snack
1 nectarine, 2 digestive cookies.	1 nectarine, 2 digestive cookies.	1 nectarine, 2 digestive cookies.	1 nectarine, 2 digestive cookies.	1 nectarine, 1 pasteli bar.	1 nectarine, 2 cream crackers.	some grapes, 2 cream crackers.
Meal	Meal	Meal	Meal	Meal	Meal	Meal
Baked omelette with 1 potato, tomato on the side, bread.	Fresh anchovies, greens, bread, tomato.	Tomato salad, pasta with minced meat sauce, cheese.	Tomato salad, burgers, 1 piece of feta cheese, bread.	Greens (a side plate), 3 – 4 meatballs, cheese, bread.	Stuffed vegetables, 2 – 3 pieces of baked potato, cheese, bread.	Grilled chicken with potatoes, tomato salad, feta cheese, bread.
snack	snack	snack	snack	snack	snack	snack
Some grapes. 1 pasteli bar.	1 nectarine, 2 cream crackers.	Some grapes, 2 cream crackers.	1 nectarine, 2 digestive cookies.	1 nectarine, 2 digestive cookies.	2 nectarine, 1 pasteli bar.	1 nectarine, 2 cinnamon cookies.

dinner	dinner	dinner	dinner	dinner	dinner	dinner
Bulgur salad with tomato and half a tin of tuna, 1 glass of wine.	2 souvlaki skewers, bread, tomato.	1 glass of milk, 2 cookies, 1 nectarine.	1 glass of milk, 2 cookies, 1 pear.	1 glass of milk, 2 digestive cookies, 1 pear.	1 pita souvlaki, some fries\ chips.	1 rusk, tomato on the side, 1 piece of feta cheese.
Physical activity	Physical activity	Physical activity	Physical activity	Physical activity	Physical activity	Physical activity
Type: - Duration: -	Type: Walking Duration: 20 mins	Type: Walking Duration: 20 mins	Type: - Duration: -	Type: - Duration: -	Type: Walking Duration: 20 mins	Type: Walking Duration: 20 mins

Observations
Very well 8/3 2010 (3/8/2010)

4.3 Key Takeaways

1. **Balance is the key:**
    - Your body thrives when you provide it with balanced, nourishing meals that include a mix of proteins, carbs, and healthy fats.
    - Starving or bingeing disrupts this balance, so aim for consistency.
2. **Listen to your hunger signals:**
    - Pay attention to when you're truly hungry versus when emotions or habits are driving you to eat.
    - Hunger is your body's natural way of communicating its needs—trust it.
3. **The importance of mindful eating:**
    - Eating slowly and savoring each bite helps you recognize fullness and enjoy your meals more.
    - Avoid distractions like screens during meals to stay connected to your body.
4. **Small, sustainable changes matter:**
    - It's not about perfection, but steady progress. Small, manageable changes in your eating habits can lead to long-term success.
    - Celebrate each positive step you take toward a healthier lifestyle.
5. **Food is not the enemy:**
    - There's no such thing as "bad" food. All foods can fit into a healthy diet when eaten mindfully and in moderation.
    - Shift your focus from restriction to nourishment.
6. **Your journey is unique:**
    - Everyone's body and path to health are different. What works for someone else might not work for you—and that's okay.
    - Trust yourself and honour your individual needs and preferences.

Chapter 5

Nutritional Intelligence

We more often inherit neuroses and illnesses from our parents than we do property.

Discovering the Nutritional Intelligence Index

5.1 Cognito ergo sum

Recently, an excellent book titled *A Manual of the Human Mind* by Polytropon editions fell in my hands. His author is Dr. Gerald Huther, a Neurobiology Professor at the University of Göttingen Psychiatric Clinic. Through numerous scientific studies, he describes how and why any person can escape various negative attitudes and tendencies from psychosomatic symptoms to negative and harmful habits that infiltrate the soul and body of the modern man. He characteristically states that the way the human brain evolves depends on its use and what has been done to it until now; what should we actually do to enable our brain to develop to its full potential?

Professor Duchess Huntett begins with the assumption that every human being has a unique mind, solely his own, that has specific inclinations and weaknesses from the first day. But what will happen during a person's life depends on whether these predispositions for better development find the right ground to develop, and whether

Nutritional Intelligence: The Answer to Bulimia, Overeating, and Obesity
Evangelos Zoumbaneas

ISBN 978-981-5129-74-8 (Hardcover), 978-981-5129-73-1 (Paperback), 978-1-003-65188-8 (eBook)
www.jennystanford.com

the proper way is discovered for existing weaknesses to be limited or overcome. It will all depend on how and for what uses each of us puts his mind to work. The place, time and environment will largely determine which of the innate skills and which of the acquired skills will be developed during their lifetime.

Until a few decades ago, there was a belief that brain development starting from infancy, stops at about the end of adolescence. That is why all the known theories persisted and rightly continue to insist on the enormous importance of the proper nurturing of children and adolescents. Very recently, it has been found that the brain, even during adulthood, is highly malleable. While nerve cells cannot divide after birth (with some exceptions), they are capable of adapting their complex interfaces to new conditions of use throughout their lives. For example, in people who were hit in the head and have lost their memory due to the destruction of brain cells, the brain itself activated other brain cells by creating new neuronal connections to restore lost memory. Also, in people crippled in their right hand, the brain soon developed new neural connections that allowed them to utilize their left hand, adopting all the skills that the right hand had until then, even skills like calligraphy.

Given that the first neuronal connections develop in early childhood and are actively integrated into later life, the most important experiences a person can gain in the course of his life are of a psychosocial nature. This means that for all the decisions we make, what drives us is not our spirit or our conscience, nor the knowledge we have gained from dubious sources, but the experiences we have had hitherto. Experiences firmly established in every person's mind shape their expectations, draw their attention to precise directions, and determine how they evaluate what they are experiencing and how they respond to what is happening in their surroundings.

5.2 I Am Therefore I Feel

Until recently, it was assumed that the brain's main use is thinking. Still, all current findings have shown that the human brain is primarily active in the direction of functions summed under the term "psychosocial skills." That is to say, our mind is more a social than a reasoning organ. After all, in recent years, there has been much talk of "emotional IQ" rather than plan "IQ," which, according to many studies, does not necessarily lead to a balanced and "happy" life. So, the emotions play the most significant role in the impression and recording of early experiences in the brain, in the orientation of the processes of perception and thought, and the subsequent shaping of life attitudes and beliefs.

The way one feels thinks and acts has a physical, neurobiological basis. This structure depends on the successful or incomplete development of neuronal and synaptic connections within the brain. The impressions and images recorded during our infancy during brain development still remain in our brains today as a form of recorded information somewhere in a neuronal interface. That is, all the information and knowledge available in our brains is nothing more than a neural interface. These existing neuronal connections define and characterize what we are today: our skills and weaknesses, our way of thinking, and our behaviour. Simply put, all this is nothing more than a reflection of how our one and only mind works.

5.3 Sins of Parents, Relatives, Teachers, Politicians, Ministers of Education Are Passed on to Children

The most common reason why sometimes our minds lead us to react negatively in certain situations by amplifying various disorders is based on severe mistakes usually made from very early on. These mistakes mainly stem from the period when our parents and other individuals of our close social environment are those who determine how and why the mind is used. Later in school, the circle of those who influence our perception is further expanded. The way we use our minds is greatly influenced by the perceptions of 'third parties' that we come across. And if you consider that the world and environment that a child comes into and is brought up within is, more or less, built on the norms and beliefs of previous generations, then we really have to rethink whether this environment in which we have lived until now was the most favourable for the development of a human mind. The less these conditions are met, the more mistakes will be made, and the more disorders will the developing generation inevitably incorporate in its mental function.

The more unilateral and incomplete inputs a brain receives during its developmental phase, the more often the individual will apply some very specific destructive strategies each time difficult conditions are encountered. Such conditions cause feelings like stress, sadness, anxiety, phobias, anger, etc. This results in the person reacting impulsively and reflexively without evaluating the actual magnitude of the situation they have found themselves involved in, additionally failing to recognize the very feelings that have triggered this immediate and usually self-destructive reaction. For example, the calming effects of eating food are often used against fear or stress. Frequent repetition of such behaviour results in permanent neuronal connections in the brain that eventually lead to food dependence, such as those in bulimia and anorexia. The same is true of alcohol or drugs or sedatives that, under similar conditions, either have a calming effect on the person taking them or cause euphoria and lead to addiction.

5.4 One Man, Two Minds

Psychologist Dennis Clovis in his book *Emotional Intelligence* (ed. Ellinika Grammata) claims: "We have two minds: one that thinks and one that feels. These two fundamentally different forms of knowledge interact to shape our mental existence. The rational mind is the way to understand through which we become aware: it is more conscious, thoughtful, capable of weighing situations, and thinking. But right next to it, there lies another system of knowledge, impulsive and powerful, though sometimes absurd, the emotional mind. Usually, there is a balance between the emotional and the rational mind as emotions feed and shape the rational mind's functions. The latter then refines and sometimes vetoes emotions and avoids possible negative and forced reactions. The emotional mind is a weapon of survival for every human being. For example, in the face of danger, the feeling of fear created will hasten our reactions so that we can fight or escape. In this case, it acts as a primitive reflexive instinct purely for defensive reasons. It provides a raw emotional response. But it works identically when the data has to do with all other emotional information, which concern emotions created by situations that cause anger, anxiety, panic, sadness, weakness; the emotional mind gets the upper hand subduing the rational one. Every time intense emotional information floods the brain, it is first channelled to the emotional mind as a whole. At that moment, all the conditions are created for an immediate emotional - reflective reaction. Reasonable processing of this intense information requires extra time for analysis and rationalization.

Until this is done, the intense "feeling" has already caused the emotional mind to become stimulated.

The word emotion has the word "motion" as the second constituent, and movement causes an immediate "reaction" to what is happening.

The word "reaction" contains the word "action" and this, in turn, leads directly to "impulse".

It is the impulse that ultimately determines a person's spontaneous behaviour to what is happening to him, leading him to uncontrollable reactions such as binge eating, smoking, alcohol and drug use, over-consumption of food, gambling and very often, even violence.

The latter, violence, as a final result of the exacerbation of an incorrectly rationalized feeling, has been recorded as the cause of countless offences. Crimes and acts of violence performed "in the heat of anger" by later repentant perpetrators who were certainly motivated by a bad evaluation, followed by a thoughtless reaction to a strong emotion.

5.5 The Secret Plan: "Code: Stop"

If before every person reaches the "stimulation" stage, that is to say, instead of simply acting on the impulse, he had the ability and patience to wait a few moments for the situation to also be evaluated by the rational mind before deciding on which the most appropriate reaction would be, numerous unpleasant situations would have been avoided. Some instant, direct commands to the brain itself such as "calm down and think before acting", "think of alternatives", "think about the consequences in advance", "talk about the problem and how you feel about it", "you don't have to find all the alternatives on your own"," go ahead and try the best plan", would be very useful.

It takes will to keep emotions under control. The time required for the emotion to reach its peak is too short, it only takes a few seconds. The rational mind takes just a few seconds more than its emotional counterpart to record events and react to them. Psychologist Daniel Goleman states that the first impulse belongs to the heart and not the mind. If this small "pause before reacting" is achieved then there will be a second kind of emotional reaction, slower than the immediate one, which is underlying and starts forming in our thoughts before we reach the impulsive emotional response. That is to say, the whole game is won when thought precedes the impulsive reaction created by a strongly negative feeling. If one also manages to clarify what exactly the emotion is that drives him to some adverse reaction each time, then the path to a more balanced life based on sensible and beneficial decisions will also be opened. Of course, the latter is not the easiest thing to achieve, especially for people suffering from some kind of disorder. Usually, a lot of knowledge, a great deal of self-awareness, and certainly a small, or big help from a psychotherapist are required. I think it's a huge waste of time - if not a whole life wasted - until someone learns to recognize and express their true feelings about it and the help of a psychotherapist will surely help save valuable time. A personal problem is always well hidden in every eating disorder. The big question is, when we uncover the fault in nutrition, what happens with the underlying issue? As psychologist Danai Colette describes very characteristically, "emotional self-awareness becomes the cornerstone for the next building of emotional intelligence, that is, the ability to get rid of a bad mood."

5.6 Am I Sad, Angry, or Hungry?

Individuals who are unable to distinguish and control depression symptoms are usually potential victims of eating disorders. When this is combined with an intense dissatisfaction with body image, the next step is usually either bulimia nervosa or anorexia nervosa. Also, many people fail to distinguish between being scared, angry, and hungry, so they combine all these feelings into one: the feeling of hunger that drives them to overeat whenever they are stressed or anxious.

When the habit of calming oneself by eating after an emotional storm meets the stress of staying thin, then an eating disorder is already present. At first, one can eat obsessively but then, to stay slim he may vomit, start taking laxatives, or stop eating altogether. For one, getting rid of these destructive habits is not as simple as finding someone who speaks with the voice of reason, telling him that he must stop because he is hurting himself. Once a person is already in the grip of an eating disorder, the real solution will come only after he first learns to recognize his feelings. After learning to calm himself and on the necessary condition that he manages to better handle the relationships with the people around him - whether they are members of his family or otherwise closely related with constant and daily interaction. But if these people had learned during their childhood to openly express and recognize their feelings before they were inflicted with an eating disorder, if they had learned to state clearly that they were hungry, bored, sad, scared, they would not have a problem not only with eating disorders but also many other aspects of their lives. In the same way, we, the older ones, should speak openly when we talk to our children or meet other people: "Now I'm angry about what you did," "I am sad at the moment," "I am happy", "I am proud of you" "you are very beautiful" and why not every time before falling asleep "I love you so much". If you do not express your feelings, how will you be able to recognize them? After all, "everything that is not put into words... is put into the body".

5.7 Decoding the Emotion

People who feel confident in their emotions manage their lives better and gain a more down-to-earth sense and awareness of the decisions they make for themselves. Emotional self-control, the subjugation of our impatience and the nurturing of impulsivity lie above all achievements. People who have this ability tend to be much more productive and effective with whatever they deal. For example, recognising that "what I feel now is anger" offers a greater degree of freedom, not only by preventing it from influencing our actions, but it also allowing ourselves to try to get rid of it. Every time we pause before the next impulsive step to which we have been led by a feeling, our brain develops a new neuronal interface, stores new information in its own cells, acquires the ability to meditate, and learns to restraint itself. Each next stop for meditation and meditation builds an extra-neural connection and reinforces previous ones. With each subsequent one they all end up rooting over the last imperfect interconnections, eventually restoring the coveted balance.

Therefore, it is important to change the current conditions that lead us to dead-end paths so that the new ones will enable us to develop new skills and new visions by changing our brain function.

The search for those interconnections responsible for the spiritual, social, or the family environment in which one is born is, after all, rather meaningless. Only in one thing can it be useful for each of us to become aware of how they act in shaping a particular climate so as not to make the same mistakes. Since the environment in which we will grow up and live in the future can also change, just like the way we will use our minds from one point on.

5.8 I Am an Adult and Now I Decide for Myself

How we use our brains from one time on will determine our future. Whether we stay in the current situation or move on gaining new skills and implementing better practices depends on the personal attitude we choose to pursue. Once we know that we can attach new neuronal connections, we can "reprogram" our brains. As Professor Dr Gerald Huther says, the human brain can overwrite old interconnections with new formations, remodel and replace them, and alter old patterns of reasoning and behaviour even if they are seemingly fundamental beliefs and emotional structures. Therefore, it is possible for even adults to repair possible unilateral, anomalous or incomplete brain areas that were formed during the developmental phase of the brain.

The aim of corrective interventions is to restore the lost internal balance. The key to any fresh start is to recognize that a problem exists. That is, to recognize that some of the actions one has performed so far lead to nowhere – apart from self-destruction - to motivate the individual to find solutions and get people to help him get rid of the vicious circle of an established state, or situation. After all, a Chinese proverb says that "if you recognize what the problem is, then you can find a solution."

In this chapter, we will study how to use the knowledge provided by neurobiology to more easily apply all of what has been described, to work out a tactic one must follow to get rid of an eating disorder. The phrase of Professor Gerald Huther that "our minds are lifelong educable and life-changing" is characteristic.

5.9 Neurobiology in the Service of Treating Eating Disorders

Suppose you have a desire to do something completely new. If, for example, today you take some balls and start being a juggler, you will force your mind to continuously develop skills in coordinating motions until you can simultaneously maintain control of several balls. If today you decided to walk on a narrow wood plank and day by day you reduced its surface, the brain would develop new neuronal connections giving you the ability to balance even on a stretched rope. And if you realized your desire to become a botanist tomorrow, soon even the shortest walk in the countryside would turn into reconnaissance trip for hundreds of different species of shrubs and flowers. So, unlike all other living beings, man can freely decide how he wants to use his mind and how he wants to shape it. The mere fact that a person can train his mind to perform for a chosen purpose is enough to prove that the brain can adapt to functions required of it.

5.10 The Right Moment and the Necessary Time

"Where there is a will, a new path is revealed," says Professor Dr. Gerald Huther. As for the path that should be followed to get rid of an eating disorder, again one should start from the assumption that something is wrong with himself and his diet. Deciding to reduce or control the intake of food, either due to remarks about gaining weight, because one is no longer accepted "the way he has become", or because one is prepared to follow a diet plan until they reach the desired weight and then returning to their old habits, are the classic components of failure. Only real awareness of the situation can program a brain to change permanently.

The minimum time required for the re-registration of all pre-existing unilateral and incorrect neuronal connections blamed for the inconvenient condition is two to five years. Only when a person adopts new eating habits, with daily exercise for at least five years, and in combination with regular weekly exercise, can they feel confident that they have reprogrammed their brain, at least in terms of nutrition and ideal body weight.

5.11 Walking on Both Legs You Get There Faster

If one visits my place of work, the first thing they will come across is a huge announcement that reads: "No diet plan guarantees any results unless it is accompanied by physical activity." When you desire to change your body weight to finally reach your goal, you will have walk there on both "legs": One is nutrition, and the other exercise. You can't get anywhere on one "leg" alone. Neither only with diet, nor just with exercise. Not even sometimes using a little more of the one and other times the other. A very typical phrase I use when I meet people who want to lose weight just by correctly following their diet is "indeed, you have a very good left leg; though, it would be far better if you improved your right one too" implying the importance of both to achieve the goal—proper nutrition and exercise on a daily basis.

5.12 Stop Being a Fan of the SCB (Sofa Chair Bed)

The best mindset to help people with weight problems is to think that their day should no longer have 24 hours. It should be 23 hours long, and the remaining hour should be devoted to a simple daily walk, or any other form of physical activity. Even playing with your kids, taking them out for a stroll, taking advantage of the waiting time to pick them up from their afternoon activities, walking to work or getting off the bus three stops earlier, etc. One excellent assumption is that "television is seriously detrimental to health unless you are on a treadmill". Once this has become part of your mentality, you will be surprised by the possibilities and opportunities that you will come up with in order to exercise.

5.13 When the Weighing Scale Blinds You and You Don't See the Results

"Don't worry about your weight, but what you eat." Experience here has repeatedly confirmed that people who have improved their eating habits without ever undergoing a hypocaloric diet, inserting an hour of daily, low intensity exercise into their program, slim down without any further effort. Relieved of the stress caused by constant weighing and with the only monitoring criterion being the changes in their body, have succeeded in obtaining such extraordinary changes in their appearance that they have become a permanent boasting subject. Following a plan of adequate nutrition and regular physical activity are followed by an unexpected change in their physical characteristics that often come in complete contrast with the results of weighing. There are innumerable examples of people continually changing sizes of clothes in stark contrast to the weighing scales' results, showing no more than a little weight loss after one month. Still, the physical changes were proportional to a lot more than that. In the end, all these people feeling good about their bodies, was and will be the essence of the whole matter.

The big problem that all nutrition scientists face is how to clean the "garbage" that has accumulated on the heads of each of our clients for years. Trash like "If I can't lose a pound a week, then diet is wrong." "If I'm 1.60 in height and I'm not 50kg, then I'm still fat." Garbage that has been stacking higher with every weighing on the weighing scales for years and continue to do so. Feeling good about your body, wearing what you like, and flattering yourself is better than having one or two million euros in your bank account. The point is being happy with what you have. Regular exercise, along with proper nutrition, can generously provide you with the "aesthetic wealth" you need.

5.14 Objective: Before You Go Hungry Don't Be Hungry, and Before You Are Thirsty Don't Go Thirsty

The nutrition program described at the end of Chapter 4 with the three primary and properly combined meals and the two in between, can only work if one uses it as a remedy against bulimia and binge eating. Food should be consumed on a schedule, with the maximum time between meals being no more than 2.5 to 3 hours. This is when the nutrients from the previous meal will be depleted and the next one should start.

5.15 All That Which Have Happened for Me, in My Absence

Most of the time, we do not realize the attitudes and perceptions formed within us, nor how much we are compelled to use our minds in a particular way. When a child has watched his parents rush out of bed each morning, this has caused a permanent neuronal connection in his brain. When he has seen them eating (usually at night) the sum of a day's meals, this has become a neurotic connection as well. And every time the parents, because they have not prepared food or because the night inaction has overcome them, have phoned to order pizza, an extra-neural connection has again been created. Every time a toddler's birthday party has taken place in a fast-food restaurant or in a playroom with a similar menu, or when a family's outing has started and ended in a restaurant, then an extra-neural interconnection has been established and added to the existent ones to create a strong mesh of deep-rooted negative eating behaviours.

5.16 An Index of Nutritional Intelligence

We are bombarded, almost daily, with information on the importance of proper nutrition and the great need to change our eating habits. Knowing what is terrible and what is beneficial regarding nutrition should, in theory, have motivated everyone to aim for a better quality of life through proper nutrition. Those who have occasionally dieted and especially those who have had the right judgement to obtain their nutritional guidance through a qualified nutritionist, clearly have had the opportunity to enrich their knowledge with the most appropriate advice and information. Why does Greece still rank among the countries with the highest rates of childhood and adult obesity in Europe and in the world as a whole? Why has so much knowledge from dietitians yet to be put to use, and thousands of people break their diet and return to their old eating habits on a daily basis? For some reason, information isn't targeted and used accordingly and properly; instead, it is filtered and only a minuscule amount manages to reach all these people.

For example, whenever a dietitian advises on and explains to his client the importance of a morning meal, the information may be travelling directly from him to the client's brain, but it manages to reach him completely weakened, without really affecting him but for, perhaps, a minimum time. What is it that has happened?

Along the course this particular information crossed between the dietitian and the client, it was forced through a vast emotional net and had to be filtered through a packed behavioural grid that has remained entrenched in the mind of the client for years. How can he, in a moment, do away with a memory engraved in his mind many years ago, of his father rushing out of the house every morning on an empty stomach, but at the same time etching the information that "this is what men do" on his mind? The emotional resistance of a person suffering from an eating disorder to new information and tactics is as difficult and time consuming to face as it is to train someone to climb the summit of Mt Everest. So, it is easy to conclude that people's eating behaviour is not based on what they know but on what they feel and have experienced concerning food so far.

Suppose we could summarize each person's cognitive experience with food under one general term, we could speak of a new evaluation index, namely the **"Nutritional Intelligence Index"**.

How and to what extent each person utilizes their knowledge of nutrition behaviour can now be assessed based on the Nutritional Intelligence Index.

This indicator will express and measure:

- the skills and abilities of each person based on how they manage their daily diet,
- their level of involvement, according to their mental state and
- their ability to continue practicing good eating habits after many years.

Before, at least, two years have passed, even the best customers who strictly follow their dietitian's plan, will break their diet in the first adverse situation that will occur. A sickness in the family, a death, a change in the work environment, a break-up, a pregnancy or any other stressful situation, will trigger a disaster. On the contrary, people who have stuck to a well-chosen and organized diet for many years, have developed a mighty Nutrition Intelligence Index that helps invent alternative solutions even in the most difficult situations, or at least, brings them back to their regular and tested eating habits.

5.17 The Advantage of Being Able to Say "Enough"

For a person to return to a past state, not only of innocence but also the ability to say "enough", their diet must start again, almost from scratch. And if not from scratch, at least based on the frequency and variety of meals a child has between the ages of three and four. It is the age when parents may have the last chance to teach their children a set of proper eating habits. To do that not by saying what "must be done", but with their individual behaviour, being the first to set a good example. It is hilarious - and tragic at the same time - when an overweight parent brings his child to the dietitian to lose weight. With their personal behaviour and dietary choices, parents are solely responsible for the Nutrition Intelligence Index that will be passed on to their children.

The age between three and four years of age, is the first period in which children develop speech skills and can openly express feelings and preferences. Moreover, suppose they are fortunate enough to have small and regular meals, they also have the ability to say "enough" even if the world's most delicious food is presented. Remember or ask what a child's diet is like between the ages of three and four. Milk in the morning, breakfast later at home or in kindergarten, after two hours comes lunch, in the afternoon yoghurt with some fruit or juice, and finally, dinner: At least five meals that provide the basis to say "enough."

As soon as they go to school, the negative influences come up, such as drinking a glass of milk in a hurry and leaving for school without having breakfast and turning to the school canteen and its horrid food options to satisfy their hunger. It is precisely the moment that all previous balances will be disrupted, if a proper nutrition education hasn't yet been established and a high enough Nutritional Intelligence Index is not already present, and a life of consuming fatty and low-quality food will start.

Therefore, harmonious coexistence with food is essential not only for people with any form of eating disorder, but all people as well. Food choices should be made based not on their caloric content, but their nutritional value. When food continually offers a variety of nutrients, the body will use them to build and maintain physical and mental balance. A common example I use to explain the importance of the differentiation of foods, in contrast to the classic question of whether it is fattening or not, is the following: 'Two tablespoons of a mixture of fruits and nuts may have the same number of calories as a croissant, but the difference is that the calories from the mixture will be utilized through the transfer of all the nutrients they contain to the body, such as vitamins, minerals, amino acids, essential fatty acids etc. On the other hand, the calories from the croissant will be stored in the form of fat in the abdomen or the area around the waist.

5.18 The Solution to Craving for Sweets

For those who have followed diet plans, the instructions are clear: apply this diet and do not deviate even a bit. The treatment of eating disorders is about the opposite. "First eat all that your body needs to restore its balance, and then whatever else you wish." For example, if you want to eat a sweet in the afternoon, eat your fruit and snack, and then eat the sweet. This way you either won't need the sweet or you will eat just as much as you need to enjoy it, avoiding the addition of a second or third serving, which will lead to a bulimic episode, guilts, dieting, deprivation of food and the same all over again. "Between the options of eating less than what I know is good for me to also have a sweet or eating both the meal and the sweet, we always choose the latter." Better more by providing the nutrients that the disordered body needs than the deprivation that will lead directly to a new eating disorder relapse. After all, those who have tried to deprive themselves of proper food are well aware of this tactic's consequences: more weight, different dieting, more serious disorder.

5.19 Diet Is Like Finances: If You Do Not Make Predictions, You Will Go Broke...

Even if one does not feel hungry when he or she must eat one of the planned meals, they should consume at least a minimal amount. For example, suppose they are not hungry to eat an apple and a cereal bar at the scheduled breakfast time, they should eat at least one grape or cherry and an almond or walnut to continue controlling the biological clock of hunger. Even if one misses any critical fruit or snacks in-between meals, they should consume them a few minutes before their next main meal. It is essential to maintain balance. It is of the utmost importance to reinforce the new neuronal connections that have begun to emerge. The basic consideration to bear in mind is: "Every time we lose even one of our scheduled meals, for every new neuronal interface created when we get a regular meal, at least two of the desirable connections we have managed to create will unfortunately collapse under the weight of all the bad connections from our past eating behaviour.

The most tremendous success for a student who learns a foreign language, such as English is to learn to think directly in that language. Our obligation as nutrition scientists is to teach people to think in the language of nutrition. When one has been able to control himself and resist for more than five years all that has hitherto seduced him, then all the necessary mechanisms that will alert him to his actual food needs have been re-established in his body. A high Nutritional Intelligence Index will have been achieved when proper nutrition has become regular without people negotiating what to eat, when to eat, and even what not to eat. Just like when one wakes up in the morning and out of habit, the first thing to do is wash their face and teeth, then head mechanically to the table to have breakfast and leave the house having prepared the snack one will eat a few hours later. Indeed, many researchers believe that a person who has long adopted healthy eating habits combined with regular exercise has acquired the unique ability to know the exact amount of food their body needs in a day, down to the last calorie. Also, if one works out regularly, their body acquires an extra ability to maintain body weight even if the individual happens to consume four times the amount of food their body needs.

5.20 Will Depletes

A recent publication in the journal "New scientist" of a study by psychologists at Florida State University reported that every time a man tries to resist temptation, he also loses some of his stored power for restraint. For example, a person who follows a specific diet and often faces the dilemma of whether or not to eat a sweet and break his or her diet, exhausts a little of their reserves each time. The more often one faces such temptations, the more certain it is that they will soon overcome their inhibitions. The researchers concluded that "every time we exercise our self-control, we use little of our stored willpower, and it takes some time for our reserves to fill up again." This may explain the fact that most people who are following a hypocaloric diet for the first time usually apply it more consistently. At the same time, each subsequent attempt becomes increasingly difficult. In the same study, the researchers came to another conclusion: Individuals who had consumed natural juice shortly before the impending "resistance exercise" exhibited a much greater ability to resist than those who had consumed a sugar substitute or nothing at all. Glucose contained in natural juice, was a critical factor in increasing the levels of temperance in the face of the alluring sweet. Finally, the researchers came to yet another conclusion: Continued self-restraint reduces glucose reserves in the brain, so if there is no sustained supply of glucose from natural sources such as fruits and natural juices, it is only a matter of time before it is depleted, leading with mathematical accuracy to a vicious cycle of binge-eating episodes, guilt and interruption of diet.

5.21 Exercises of Courage and Will

To improve one's will and temperance, one must practice it just as he would his muscular system in a gym. Adopting timely fixed meals, as described above is the first step in developing a concrete eating consciousness. Introducing a specific time for exercise, for example, every afternoon at 6 pm will create a new neuronal interface that will relieve the daily dilemma of when to exercise or prevent exercise altogether, leaving more will power to be utilized for other possible dilemmas. If the goals are accurate and not blurry or general, the chances of achieving them will increase. It is better to have a positive outcome in mind than to deal with the fear of failure. Visualizing and focusing on a positive result is the best strategy towards achieving a goal.

5.22 Nutrition Is a Journey towards the Ideal Body

Proper diet, always accompanied by daily exercise, is the means for everyone to achieve their ideal body form for which they will feel proud. After all, everyone's ideal body is that with which one feels comfortable and is not defined through any kind of weighing, measuring or fashion standard. Throughout my twenty-year-long experience helping people to losing weight, I have met many more happy women with some extra weight compared to those who were thin. Nutrition aimed towards the perfect body is indeed a journey. One that you will have to fill with knowledge and experience. It is a path that will grant you the right to deviate a little to get to know some of the exquisite flavours that will come along your journey, as long as you always remember what your final destination is. If you often lose yourself to one direction or the other, you'll soon lose your orientation altogether, and returning will be increasingly tricky and will go through tough paths that may exhaust you. Allowing yourself a nice treat because you are not feeling well one day, but having eaten your afternoon meal first, believe me, matters little. Consuming more during a night out with friends, but on the assumption that you will not be entirely on an empty stomach by that time, is not a disaster.

Eating more now and then for whatever reason is also within the framework of a proper diet. As long as you forget the tale that has been told to you for so many years that, by eating anything extra, your diet is ruined. All you need to say to yourself is "what is done is done, I enjoyed it, I did it because I needed it at that moment, but right after this I am on my way again, making the right choices that will support me in completing my journey. One that will allow me to practice proper eating habits until the last day of my life". If Ithaca is the goal for the perfect body, achieving a high Nutritional Intelligence Index will be the journey.

5.23 Coffee and Cake for Breakfast in the Memorial Service of Diet

If anyone has come to read all this information and believes that their own problem or that of their client will be solved by avoiding breakfast, skipping snacks and in-between meals, minimizing meal combinations, or insisting on low-calorie diets then I'm sorry, but they have wasted their time. I also regret the time that every person who suffers from bulimia or binge eating will waste during their life. Most of all, I regret that they will continue to be a victim of considerable exploitation by all those on his way: Magic diets, blood group diets, intolerance test diets, expensive filters, "super" pills, uncomplicated surgery, detoxification clinics, celebrity diets, celebrity dietitians are always waiting for the right victim to pray upon, both mentally and financially.

"Recklessness is an attitude that does not require much thought" says Professor Dr. Gerald Huther. Anyone who manages to avoid acting recklessly from now on, will automatically need to connect and activate representations, data and events in their minds as well as consider all data before making decisions. In simple terms he will give it more thought than someone who still treats himself and those around him with recklessness and frivolity. Thought will always be a very essential measure for the preservation and maintenance of the human mind. Proper use of our minds provides the unique power that will set us free from habits and situations that waste our time and energy by allowing us to harness the whole of the potential to change how we view and utilize our surrounding society. As the teacher and author Sevi Vatala often says, "It is not only enough to love what you do, you must also love the people to whom what you do is addressed to." No use of any human mind is meaningful unless it works towards the common good of the world through processes that promote sustainable development to deliver a better future for our children and the future generations.

5.24 Summary

This book began with the story of a woman who wanted to share her story to showcase that bulimia is a problem that must stop being hidden behind taboos and social barriers. The tale of Evi is the story of the woman next door who fights with her body and food daily. Recording her story and the way we worked together was the opportunity to finally come to some conclusions that would trigger further conversation and discussion so as to help more women experiencing the same problem with food. Conversation, dialogue, acceptance of the problem on the proper basis and considerations on alternative approaches will always be the first step that every woman and a man suffering from an eating disorder, as well as every therapist seeking solutions should follow. While recording the preceding information, there was a constant dialogue and feedback on my thoughts with my colleague Ioanna Kontele. I met her when, at the age of 15 back then, she came to my office and together we created her diet plan just before she became a gymnastics champion. She had already begun getting into an eating disorder through her coaches' stifling pressure to keep her body weight very low. With my help, she was able to achieve an ideal body weight and get rid of the disorder. She has since loved the science of Nutrition. Today, she is one of the most outstanding dietitians in Greece with the highest recognition of being the Scientific Associate of the Adolescent Health Unit of Aglaia Kyriakou Children's Hospital. Through her ingenious insights and creativity, her help was especially important in completing the work you are holding in your hands. When this book was finished, I asked her to give me her insight for the last time before publishing it. Instead of calling me, as usual, she took the time to write down her overall conclusions and thoughts.

This book is really dedicated to women. Just like it began, inspired by the story of one woman, I would like it to end with the perspective of another —the view and conclusions of woman and my colleague, Ioanna Kontele.

5.25 The Closing Goes to Ioanna...

Dear Vangelis,
Although I may have, more or less, been familiar with the subject you are dealing with and having read some excerpts from time to time, this is the first chance I have had to see a complete record of your thoughts. Reading your book now, looking into it form a different perspective, I would like to share my conclusions and thoughts...

1. *My primary conclusion is that it's amazing how blessed we are. God gave us the most expensive tool in the world, our body, and he simply let us manage it ourselves.*

   It is amazing that he has bestowed upon it the gift of changing according to the circumstances, to survive and evolve. Think about how many animal species have gone extinct, and we continue evolving simply because we are educatable and malleable.
2. *As it seems, our minds, as well as our bodies have the ultimate purpose of maintaining homoeostasis. An eating disorder is one way to reach homoeostasis. For example, if a person did not use food as a source of relief at some point, he might reach the point of having a stroke due to the accumulated stress. My view is that the brain can choose to connect the same information with two different neuronal connections, one "healthy" and one "disrupted." If it chooses the healthy one you will go out for a drink with your friends after a break-up, but if it chooses the disturbed one, you will open the fridge. It is clearly a matter of choice, and we always have at least two options. Choosing the right one merely requires education and experience. The disorder is probably related to more primitive situations and is, therefore, easier to connect to such occurrences. For instance, when cave people found food, they ate it all at once because they might not find more for a week. If the brain had chosen the "do not eat any more" command, we would have simply died and gone extinct like the dinosaurs. So, having options is good for us.*
3. *Having an eating disorder is not a curse; it is a huge opportunity to become a better person. If I hadn't had a bad relationship with food at some point, I wouldn't have gotten over it and wouldn't have learned such beautiful things. We have to tell our clients that having an eating disorder presents them with an opportunity to learn something and become better. After some months, they will never worry about their weight and diet again. Think that most of those who will read your book will be people with eating disorders. They will have the opportunity to learn that they have a low "Nutritional Intelligence Index", fight to improve it, and even achieve the optimum score and feel proud for this. Those who do not have an eating disorder will not have the opportunity to learn all these beautiful things.*

4. *I have the following questions:*
    - *Would a woman have a nocturnal binge-eating episode if her husband gave her a hug for a few seconds when he returned home?*
    - *Would a child eat more if his mum gave him a hug when he was angry and asked: how are you feeling?*
    - *Would a teenage girl get into anorexia after a love disappointment if her mum had told her about the love affair she had when she was a teen?*

Thank you very much for giving me the honour of being the first person to read these thoughts. I appreciate it because with what I have learned, I feel that I have become a better person.

5.26 Key Takeaways

1. **The Importance of Nutritional Intelligence**: It is the key to understanding how your food choices impact your physical and mental health. It's not just about what you eat, but also how and why you choose it.
2. **Mindful Eating**: The idea that food is not just energy, but also an experience. Focus on your needs, not external pressures or societal constraints.
3. **The Influence of Emotions**: Recognize how emotions, such as stress or happiness, can affect your food choices, and learn how to manage these emotions without turning to food.
4. **Your Relationship with Food**: Creating a balanced relationship with food is essential. See food as a way to care for yourself, not as an enemy.
5. **The Power of Dietary Patterns**: Family and cultural patterns play a significant role in your food choices. Understand what influences you and decide what works best for you.
6. **Self-Observation and Awareness**: Track what you eat, when, and why. This process can help you identify patterns and make targeted changes.
7. **Small Steps, Big Changes**: Changing your eating behaviour is a process that requires time and persistence. Start with small, sustainable changes.
8. **Nutritional Intelligence as a Journey**: Treat this process as a continuous learning experience. Every small step is part of the journey toward health and well-being.

Chapter 6

Letters and Food for Thought

It is often that weight stays the same when what happens around us remains the same.

6.1 Letters

In this chapter, we will comment on some letters that have reached us, either through the *Diatrofi. Health & Wellness* journal, or via email to the Scientific team of "Diatrofi" at: www.diatrofi.gr. These are some of the most frequently asked questions representative of all people dealing with diet. Their letters express their constant anxiety about losing excess weight, and it is worthwhile to comment on how some useful answers are provided. Responses aimed not only at informing but also reassuring all these desperate people.

1st letter

Cell number 53

> *First of all, I would like to congratulate you on this beautiful web page. What I want to ask has to do with my eating habits. I'm 1.63, and I currently weigh 58 kg; my body fat ranges from 20% to 21%. I usually follow a healthy diet and exercise a lot.*
> *However, I am still obsessed with my weight and do not feel comfortable at 58 kg of weight. I have been trying to reduce my*

Nutritional Intelligence: The Answer to Bulimia, Overeating, and Obesity
Evangelos Zoumbaneas

ISBN 978-981-5129-74-8 (Hardcover), 978-981-5129-73-1 (Paperback), 978-1-003-65188-8 (eBook)
www.jennystanford.com

body weight to 53 kg with a 1200 calorie diet, while also reducing my body fat to minimal levels, but from time to time I experience binge eating episodes.
What worries me is why I get these eating crises and am unable to control myself! And so, I nullify what I succeed. I can't say I'm self-destructive, excessive perhaps, and I always seek perfection according to my standards. I know so much about nutrition and what I understand is that the more I learn, the more confused I become. I finally want to stabilize my weight at 53kg, and I'm so tired. Please, how can I achieve this? I know it's all a matter of mind. Note that about 4 years ago I lost 22 pounds through a hypocaloric diet due to stress, many hours of work and over-exercising for 4 hours daily (walking and gym workout). Then, I had a burnout, and this was how my body responded. Eating the same amount of food, I started putting on weight as I had greatly reduced the amount of exercise.
Thank you so much for taking the time to read my problem.

Sincerely, Eirini

Dear Eirini,

If, as you say, you are 1.63 and weigh 58 kg with body fat ranging between 20% and 21%, and considering any value below 25% is deemed normal, you are really confused for no reason at all. On the one hand, you accept and acknowledge that you have fat levels at the lower limit of what is considered normal (below which serious health problems begin) and on the other, you insist on a "number", specifically 53. It reminds me of the Greek song titled "Cell number 33" in which the artist is imprisoned in a cell numbered "33". So, instead of realizing your prison key lies on the door, you are still locked up in a cell you have built for yourself, it's just that it is numbered "53" instead. I'm not going to analyse how weight positively changes the body image of those who work out. If you check the previous answers, the process is described in answers to other readers' questions who are trapped in their own number as you are. I hope you have already started to understand what I mean. You would earn more if you compromised with your current number which for some reason resists your futile efforts. And even when you think you've defeated it, it will stay hidden somewhere inside you and at the first opportunity will attempt a counterattack that you will perceive as a bulimic crisis. The only way to beat it is to stop giving it any thought. It feeds on your anxiety; its strength increases every time you are locked in (in a room, or in a gym, it doesn't matter) and your diet or exercise trying to beat it; its dominance strengthens within your body and mind every time you don't go out to enjoy your life, your desires, your friends. Imagine when you are perfect and have invested time, pain, and effort into achieving it, and having met a bunch of interesting men and eavesdrop them saying to each other. "Eirini is a beautiful girl, but..." This "but" makes all the difference, and you will always be defeated in a battle between two numbers whether now that they are 58 and 53 or later that they will become 58 and 55 or 60 and 55 etc. Get out and enjoy your body which is almost perfect, just like everything which is never perfect anyway. True beauty lies in knowing how to emphasise the individual features of your body. For someone it's her hips, for someone else her breasts, eyes, humour or spirit, no matter what it is or which of them one chooses to emphasise. What matters is that we are ok with ourselves and our imperfections. The most charming people are the ones who have the courage to self-embrace, not by becoming provocative, but through their witty humour and confidence. We strive for beauty, to be attractive and passionate, but in the end, what is left of people's relationships and keeps the bond between them is emotional and spiritual communication. The key to your prison is on the door. Reach out and grab it, get rid of your fears and compulsions, and unlock your life.

2nd letter

When anorexia knocks on our door

In the period 2005-2006, I came in contact with a world invisible to me until then. Through my tenure at the Adolescent Health Unit of Aglaia Kyriakou Children's hospital, which hosts such incidents and is an excellent school for me, I found out that this is a problem that has started reaching enormous proportions in our country as well. This summer, I realized that there is an exorbitant number of young girls who are, with mathematical precision, driven to the turmoil of this disease.

Anorexia nervosa is a deep internal wound that manifests itself with disproportionate consequences on the body and mind until its existence is acknowledged by the sufferer's family and broader environment. It is not immediately and easily understood. Its effects and symptoms are only discernible when it has developed considerably and, unfortunately, many times past the point of no return.

Let's get an idea of a young woman's personal experience as she described it to us in a letter that we received.

> *Love your body...*
>
> *Good morning. I am 20 years old and since I became 19, I have had nutritional problems. First it was anorexia nervosa and then bulimia nervosa. At first, my weight was average to slim at (118-132) pounds of weight at 1.75cm of height, and then, in a relatively short time, I lost a lot of weight and reached 112 pounds. You understand that I was too thin, so much so that my menstruation was interrupted for some months. From that point on, anorexia began to alternate with bulimic episodes and become more and more frequent. From April to September, I never ate normally even once. I would either eat nothing for 3 or 4 days or ate everything in my way. I had tried vomiting, thankfully without success. By September, my weight had returned to its normal levels, of course, against my wishes. I weighted 58-60 kgs and my period was back, but I suffered. I wanted to lose weight no matter what. I thought I was fat. And then I went to the opposite extreme, for 2 weeks I was home eating all day. I put on 14 kilos in 2 weeks. I had reached my lowest point. Finally, I went to a psychologist with the encouragement of my family, and now after so many months, I feel better. I've started losing weight. My goal is to reach the weight I was at previously and stay there. The truth is that many times I'm afraid I won't make it, but I want to believe that I will come out victorious. I would like to make a plea to the girls and especially the younger ones to love their body the way it is, with its particularities and not forget that true beauty must be accompanied by health.*

Letters like that from Nana have reached us many times in the past. Nana accurately describes the psychological drama that thousands of young girls have gone through. In both anorexia nervosa and bulimia, the underlying causes are mostly psychogenic. A psychiatric disorder – which may be due to many different reasons - results in the creation of a distorted body image to the individual.

The psychogenic causes that remain unresolved and non-negotiable for a shorter or longer time period, push the person to exaggerated reactions. Specifically, the relief of emotional tension is incorrectly directed to the body and is either expressed through over-eating or starvation. This distortion of the image, through the brain, results in the person not balancing between what is real or proper, and the imaginary - what is desirable. Although this subject still needs much discussion to be fully analysed, we would like to focus on two or three particular points in this letter.

Firstly, it is made clear by Nana that she sought help from her psychologist before it had become clear to her that her body was the unfortunate recipient of a self-destructive mania. She clearly understood that she would need further assistance to clear up all that had confused her mind and soul.

Another essential information Nana mentions is that her period stopped at a particular weight, at which she also got it back. We would really like all the girls looking to lose more and more weight and for all those around those girls to me mindful of this fact. Period combined with the weight point at which it is lost or regained, provide a reference point for the minimum weight that a young woman is allowed to reach. Below that, loss of period is a given, and the negative effects on the individual's health, if this persists for a long time period, are almost irreparable.

When weight is reduced to just one gram below that of the last period, growth in adolescent girls is interrupted, large organ groups such as the liver, heart and kidneys decompose, bone degradation begins with depravation from calcium, increasing the chance of osteoporotic fractures and the brain significantly reduces its functions, reaching even to the point of complete lack of communication with its environment.

This is "point zero," which should in no way be crossed and is completely distinct for any young woman. This determining weight must be continuously monitored and maintained, providing a steady and monthly period with a normal blood flow of about five days.

The role of the dietitian as a health professional and scientist, is to take into consideration the medical history and clinical condition of the individual, and in a responsible way, help the patient not to lose more weight and reverse the course of the disorder. However, there are plenty of "dietitians" who are profit-focused and are willing to suggest any form of diet, as long as their client wants it, ignoring all the dangerous side effects.

In any such case, the role of the dietitian is to first prevent the upcoming consequences that come with loss of menstruation and guide the young woman to reach the appropriate weight so that her female physical functions may come back to normal.

Then through contact, conversation, and the relationship of trust which will develop, the dietitian will, in the most pleasing way, train the young woman to acquire good eating habits, of course, always with the psychological support of a qualified psychologist.

Finally, we would like to focus on Nana's last phrase, a plea to all young girls, and I would simply like to repeat her words. **"I would like to make a plea to the girls and especially the younger ones to love their body the way it is with its particularities and not forget that true beauty must be accompanied by health"**. We totally agree with you Nana, and we really thank you for your letter and the opportunity to comment on such an important issue.

3rd letter

When the weighing scales stop going down

I'm just 21 years old, I weigh 65 kg, I have a height of 1.57m, and I do not work out. I have a severe problem with my appearance, I have very intense cellulitis, and everyone calls me "fat". I don't know what to do, at times I've started running and cycling, but I gave up because I didn't see any results. It is challenging to follow a diet because my recent medical examinations showed that my haematocrit was 35, and now I take iron supplements. What do you advise me to do to build up my self-image and my psychology?

Dear Stephania,

Proper nutrition combined with exercise can clearly produce results. But there are two important things to keep in mind. When you say you can't follow a diet, that doesn't mean you should eat uncontrollably or without planning. Clearly, there should be organized meals in your diet including a good nutritious breakfast, a well-balanced lunch, a light dinner and, of course, two intermediate meals or fruit snacks and a small snack. Also, it takes time and patience to see results in the gym. Keep in mind that people who exercise may have less weight loss but definitely present a greater change in reducing their overall body mass. The body undergoes a redistribution, and the end result justifies those who exercise. Proper nutrition and exercise are the keys to your success, but it also requires some patience.

4th letter

Is it the food or the reasons for which we eat that makes us bigger?

> *Hi, my name is Helen, and I am 41 years old. I have been visiting a dietitian regularly for 8 years.*
> *Every time I go, he gives me a new program. But my problem is NOT the diet, but the reason that makes me eat uncontrollably, especially at night.*
> *Why do dietitians think that a diet will help the patient? Is it the food we eat or the reasons why we eat? Why isn't there any help for these people, always under a dietitian's supervision, to reach their goal?*

Dear Helen,

The problem you are facing is not uncommon. Too many people, and unfortunately, most of them women, react in a similar way to yours. You simply have the courage to express it. Consider however that, your reliance on eating is an expression of the tension you experience every day. In the evening, when most people relax from their daily duties, they often find refuge in food. But think that if you expressed your feelings, thoughts and concerns, just as you now openly express your problem, there would probably be no need for you to decompress form all this or cover them through food.

In the traditional Greek society that we live in, it is engraved in the Greek woman's mentality to constantly serve others, meet everyone's needs, and forget to deal with her own. You know we don't always have to act as superheroes having time to take care of everything. We do not always need to be there for anyone who asks for our help. We will never be able to satisfy everyone. It's good to offer what we can, but to be able to help, we first must take care of ourselves. We don't always need to be there for anyone who ask for our help. It's not always possible to offer more than we have, but it is safer and more realistic to offer what we are able to. Don't wait for someone else to make sure of this. Clearly, in your case, either the diet or the binge eating episodes simply distract you from the deeper causes that trouble you during your daily routine.

Unfortunately for the modern Greek woman, it is as though she is forced to be impeccable in many different roles every day. This in itself causes intense stress, and keep in mind that under stress, you cannot help (not just you but no one else) and take care of yourself at the same time. Proper nutrition can help you stay on your feet, not strict diets. It would be preferable at this point to maintain a steady weight and start eating properly (avoiding or minimizing the devastating effects of dieting) until you develop new skills, find better communication formulas with people in your environment, find solutions that will distract you from eating during difficult times and people who can understand you and especially hear you loud and clear, just the way you expressed your concerns when you took the courage to write and this letter. Certainly, the care of a psychologist trained on eating disorders would help you to quickly identify the real causes that disturb your balance.

As for nutrition, don't expect miracles right now. Food can have a nutritional impact on a person's desire for food. The need for food could have psychological causes. Still, it may also be due to nutritional reasons and the lack of valuable nutrients leads to the search for food intake.

An excellent example to make this comprehensible is described below: "Whether an individual is led to a binge eating episode depends on two factors. One has to do with eating, and the other has psychological causes. Imagine that our body has to play a daily match whose end result depends on the score of two halves. Winning the first half depends on how well we are prepared on a nutritional level. If we ensure an excellent nutritional effect through the quality of our food and regular meals, then the 1st half is ours. Whether we will lose the second half due to psychological reasons, cannot be predicted at the beginning of the day. However, it is not possible to lose the second half every day because of our mental state. But if we have lost the first half because of poor nutrition, then the game is as good as lost at half-time. Unfortunately, the final defeat will be blamed as a whole to psychological reasons. So, let's win as many first halves as we can and then see how we handle the situation.

That is, even if there are binge eating episodes, let them happen after you have consumed everything you need to take care of your body. And rest assured that the more appropriately combined nutrients you put into your body, the more you will gain the physical strength to resist overeating. The better you eat, the more slowly you will begin to reduce the caloric intake from binge eating episodes. For example, today, you can have a binge eating episode of 2000 calories but tomorrow or the day after tomorrow, you will only need 1800 calories to stop eating. Next week you will need even fewer, and you will gradually begin to reduce the frequency of these episodes. And as your body gets stronger, your skills and ability to understand what's going on inside you will also improve, making you stronger every day.

That is why it is essential to understand that we will first repair your body as if it were a car and then you will be able to properly run. We will first restore the balance to the appetite and satiety mechanisms and then move on. "Then and only then will you truly be ready to complete your program and finally be able to maintain the weight you deserve.

5th letter

Whenever I look at my diet plan, I go crazy.

Hello. I'm 26 years old, 1.65m in height and weighing at 134 pounds. While watching my diet because I have lost 57 pounds with a dietitian's help, now I am going through a crisis of bulimia. Once a week I eat whatever food I can get my hands on. I have been training at least 3 times a week for the last 6 months. I have noticed that I am losing weight and when I see the diet sheet, I go crazy. I want to lose 10 pounds. I have gone to my dietitian, received a diet plan but have not been able to lose weight because of anxiety and panic. I want to weigh myself every day. I'm currently fasting. If I eat until 7 in the evening while eating less, will I be able to lose some weight? Since I have been on diet before, having lost much weight, I know what foods to choose, but do you have any suggestions for fasting (due to religious reasons)?

It is indeed frequent for people to have an increased tendency to eat after losing a lot of weight. This is justified because the body has been deprived of many nutrients for a long time due to the necessarily hypocaloric diet. A dietary supplement that contains vitamins B, Chromium and one with omega-3 fatty acids would greatly help you reduce your tendency for binge eating episodes. A breakfast that includes fresh juice or fruit, dairy, and wholegrain cereal would significantly help you control the amount of food you consume. In intermittent meals, include at least two to three fruit and two low-calorie snacks. Finally, I would suggest you refrain from dieting and start eating well within the range of a Mediterranean diet with many choices, always keeping your meals at half the quantity of a restaurant serving, accompanied by a salad of seasonal vegetables. I would also recommend avoiding daily and frequent weighing and listening more to what your body needs. There is no ideal weight but a weight range that may deviate 4 to 8 pounds. After all, as you said, you exercise regularly and may have changed the characteristics of your body, that is, you may have replaced the weight of the fat that you have lost with muscle mass so that you do not see significant differences in the weighing scales but in your clothes and, in general, your appearance, which is the goal. When it comes to fasting, it is a good idea to buy a vegetarian recipe book and visit an organic store where you will find a huge selection of foods that you can easily introduce to your diet.

6th letter

My husband is tired of dieting. What can I do?

> *Good evening, my husband is 33 years old, with a height of 1.73m and weighing 440 pounds. He has dieted many times but loses little or no weight and has gotten tired. As far as I know, my husband has no health problems or thyroid issues, but he must lose weight because judging by the body mass index, he is within the first grade of obesity. How can I help him?*

Dear friend,

Merely fact that your spouse has been on a diet many times - and is presumed to have regained the weight he has lost - proves that he should finally stop going from a strict diet to even tougher ones, and finally adopt better eating habits. I am certain he often can't wait to stop dieting to return to a lifestyle he is comfortable with, which clearly sooner or later leads to gaining weight. Sometimes, it is preferable to set a specific day and meal e.g., on Sunday at noon, when there could be a greater variety and plentifulness instead of this constant and continuous deprivation that leads your spouse to a point of rightful indignation. It should also be remembered that the more diets a person has followed, the more, in each subsequent attempt, difficult it is for them to lose weight. I would suggest you find a professional nutritionist who will design a daily healthy diet plan for your spouse as well as the whole family, that will include a variety of well-balanced meals for the three main meals of the day and include fruit snacks in-between. Finally, I would like to give you some advice about your spouse. His day should not be 24, but 23.5 hours long. What this means is that he should introduce 30 minutes of physical activity to his daily life, the simpler form of which being a thirty-minute walk or two fifteen-minute walks with some rest time in between. And clearly, weight-loss a goal should be set for the long run, and not so much regarding weight, but in circumference of the abdomen, which should reach between 90 and 95 centimetres.

7th letter

The consequences of vomiting

> *My name is Despina and recently my sister told me that every time she goes out with her boyfriend for dinner when she returns home, she vomits to avoid getting fat. I am very much concerned about this and have recently read on www.diatrofi.gr an article on eating disorders. Lately, I think she's vomiting many times per day, but my sister tells me that what vomiting is all about is not getting fat, but I think the issue is much more severe than she thinks. I have even noticed lately that she is always tired, has frequent dizziness and her teeth have changed colour, becoming yellowish and she constantly complains of nausea. I would like your advice on whether vomiting can be harmful to her health.*

Dear Despina,

We believe that your sister already suffers from bulimia nervosa, and it will likely lead to Anorexia nervosa at some point in the future. This requires a great deal of attention for this to stop as soon as possible under the supervision of specialised therapists.

The self-inflicted vomiting frequently used by your sister can have the following effects.

Causing vomiting to eliminate the food consumed results in irritation of the stomach, oesophagus and oral cavity. The stomach contains a strong acid that breaks down food. When this acid comes in contact with other parts such as the oesophagus and the oral cavity (teeth, gums, etc.) it causes irritation, tissue erosion, wounds, or inflammation. It is very likely for the individual to feel pain and a tingling sensation in the oesophagus and gums and most likely, this will have led to tooth erosion. The irritation of the oesophagus (which is sensitive to this acid) is so intense that it can cause an ulcer or rupture (open wound). Additionally, pockets are formed in the tonsils from food residue that, apart from being annoying, can also cause infection.

Electrolyte disturbances are also significant. Purging of food and stomach fluids causes a substantial loss of potassium, resulting in heart arrhythmias and hypotension, sometimes leading to a heart attack. Along with electrolytes, water is also lost, resulting in hypotension, dizziness and dehydration, so your sister feels very tired and her skin will definitely be dehydrated. All this in combination with hypoglycaemia (as glucose does not get absorbed energy into the body) can lead to fainting and loss of consciousness, very dangerous if one thinks that when fainting, one can get badly hurt.

Trying to induce vomiting is dangerous. It has been observed that the voluntary induction of vomiting creates an increase in pressure due to over-effort and because of this, vessels rapture, even a stroke.

Not absorbing the nutrients your sister's body needs for the proper function of the body depletes her physical reserves in the long run. This results in osteoporosis, avitaminosis, development of disease, and severe exhaustion. Also, there are problems with memory, attention and thought organization as all the components that help the brain function are missing. Lack of nutrients even leads to mood swings, depression and lack of interest!

It is also essential to explain to your sister that the body does not lose weight with vomiting because metabolism requires many nutrients which she deprives herself of by vomiting. Finally, due to the lack of nutrients, the body does not understand that it is full and thus hunger comes after vomiting, and after this, a bulimic episode. Then vomiting again. and you live in a vicious cycle that never ends. We advise you to share your concern about all these consequences with your sister and discuss this matter together to persuade her to seek help immediately.

8th letter

Parents failing the exams...

Dear magazine, my name is Katerina, I am an overweight mother and I have dragged my older daughter into it. Every day she faces a big problem at school with the other kids who make fun of her, which makes her feel bad, and has a negative effect on her school performance. She cannot concentrate on studying and is always jealous of my youngest daughter. Especially ever since the second child was born, it's gone too far... This year as the new school year begins and she will go to the next class, I am afraid that things will go from bad to worse. I have made countless attempts to lose weight, but none thus far has had a lasting effect. But I really want to help my child and am willing to do whatever is suggested to make it happen.

Dear Katerina,

Attending a "parenting school" will teach people things like "if they want their child to do well at school, the child should play for at least one hour every day during the first years of his life in the room where he will have to concentrate to study in the future". For example, in his room, when the crib goes out, his desk will replace it, filled with pencils, notebooks, and books. Also, to achieve this, from the age of infancy, they must spend time with him and his toys in this space, for at least one hour, the mother and the father, but on one condition. They will be busy playing with their child and nothing else. They won't use mobiles, answer the phone, the television will be off in the background. Hence, the message is that when we focus on something, we focus on it and nothing else. They also use this tactic to reinforce a feeling of trust in their child that they are unique and not part of their free time.

Attending a parent-school teaches that the older child is jealous of the new-born entering the home. What are the emotions that drive the child to react so strongly? For example, when you get a new dining table, what do you do with the old one? Do you throw it away or take it to the country house? This is how the older children feel. They are afraid their parents will neglect them. And that feeling is especially intense when, in the first days after the birth of a new member, the older child goes to live with his grandparents for a few days, literally removing him from his everyday life as if you were throwing him away. And even if parents do not remove the older child, why is the child still having jealousy symptoms? How would you feel if your spouse suddenly brought you a second spouse to live together? This is how the older child feels for a long time until he or she understands the concept of brotherhood.

Attending a parenting school teaches them why not all children fall into drugs, why they are not all led to crime, why some children succeed, and others don't. All he needs is to get the information promptly and, above all, to know how to behave from infancy to early elementary school, where most of the temperament develops during these first five to six years in every child.

In society, not all children are drawn to alcohol or drugs, or crime. They may try, and most likely they will all try, the new, strange, and extreme but some of them will stop it in time, some will control themselves and show restraint. And unfortunately for those who are or will become parents, whatever path their children take, they will be and will remain being the sole person responsible for them. Just as in an earthquake, not all buildings fall, so not all children are drawn to alcohol or drugs or crime in a society. Even if the tiles were broken after the earthquake, even if the plaster is cracked, everything is rebuilt even a collapsed roof. However, if the building's foundations have come down, it cannot be erected again. Buildings with solid foundations remain upright in every rocking and shaking of life. The stronger the foundations, the more shocks they will withstand.

Children's health is built during the first years of their lives. Whether they get good or bad eating habits depends on how others around them act. Children up to the age of five do not learn from recorded knowledge but copy what they see. And what they see will apply for most of their lives.

The new school year has just begun. You must admit that you and all of us need new knowledge since ignorance is the greatest sin and information is the best prevention. Attending a parenting school or searching for wisdom on becoming a better parent ultimately does not teach the reasons why some children will be more successful or thrive more than others. It teaches how to become a successful parent because the concept of failing a class integrates that of loss. There is now a great need to deliver a better future for our children. There is a great need to teach our children that the future belongs equally to all children of the world.

9th letter

Letter to all overweight people by an overweight individual in recovery

I have wondered many times whether being overweight is purely a matter of will. The truth is that if it were just a matter of choice, we would all be able to lose the excessive weight that is troubling us. The answer is that all of us, and all of us who have weight problems, are so eager to slim down that we consume an infinite amount of time, money, and energy in our efforts to achieve it.

The problem of obesity is so multifactorial, like the monster Hydra. You cut one head, and suddenly, two new ones appear for you to fight with. To make it, we all need to understand that our excessive weight is the symptom, not the problem. For example, when we get sick, the fever is not the problem; it is our body's defence against the virus that has invaded our body. To lose weight, we need to take some time, take a look at our lives, and identify the real reasons that caused our weight gain. It's like putting our lives under the microscope to see, for the first time and with our own eyes, the cause of the problem, the virus that has caused the disease. If we look closely, we will see that our weight depends on our psychology (how we manage our emotional stalemates), on our overall lifestyle and diet (sedentary life, poor food choices, the environment in which we live and work etc.), but also from biochemical factors (inadequate nutrition at the cellular level, hormone imbalance, insulin resistance, etc.) and maybe other factors that don't currently come to mind.

While we often have the will, we do not use the right means to accomplish our purposes. For example, I hear that many people who want to lose weight are not prepared to put exercise into their lives. However, our body is made for movement; it is made for running, climbing, walking, and generally moving. If we do not do so, we act against our nature. As we do so, we become ill and unhappy and, if we also add non-nutritious processed foods to our daily diet, such as sugar, sweets and fat-rich and saturated foods, our body will have no way of burning or discarding them and it is meant to continue starving for the nutrition we do not provide it. Even if we are on a diet and do not eat fatty foods without exercising, losing weight becomes a race against nature, a race against our body, whose food we deprive it of more than we need to. If we do not do so, we will not lose weight since we do not have a high enough metabolic rate. And I ask you, how long do you think you can voluntarily starve? How strong is your will, and how much do you think you can last, acting against your nature? A month? Two months? Not much more I reckon.

After starvation come strong survival instincts and hunger can no longer be managed. And we live in a world where a plethora of sweet, sugary and easily accessible foods. Indeed, when we starve after so much deprivation, we do not eat fruits, vegetables, or any nutritious food. Our need for something sweet (because of low blood sugar level) or something fatty (because our brains are starving) is so great that it is stronger than our will and desire to lose weight. Because hunger is our most robust resistance to death, hunger is what has helped the human species to survive until the present day, it is one of the strongest instincts of self-preservation. And I wonder when I see people nowadays dieting and getting hungry voluntarily... Where are you heading, my good fellow, totally unprepared???

My long fight with excessive weight taught me the following: There are no magic diets, magic pills, creams that will help us lose weight and inches fast, efficiently and effectively. This is a vast utopia, a "trip" into which the modern slimming industry puts us, to get its hands on a portion of our income. The harsh truth is that the only thing that will work in the long term, to lose weight but more importantly maintain this new, lower weight is changing our lifestyle and diet. Let's start to really love ourselves because only then will we care for it like it deserves. Let's start exercising not to lose weight, but to feel good and healthy. After 30 minutes of walking, everything will seem better since the stress hormones will be reduced and our minds will be clear. Whatever concerns us will be solved more efficiently. Let's start choosing nutritious and healthy food, not to lose x amount of weight in x months, but to be healthy. Let's finally learn not to "swallow" all our sorrows, anger or despair, let's learn to express ourselves, be unpleasant, and just say "no"! Let us learn to stay away from toxic people and toxic food or, if this is sometimes not possible, at least let us additionally give our body proper nutrition and exercise so it can discard toxins.

And if all of that seemed unattainable to me at first, I thought the secret lies in small increments of change rather than large ones. The smoother we move to a healthier lifestyle the easier we will be able to maintain it for a lifetime. We cannot become another person from one day to the next; transformation is a

time-consuming process. Personally, I like seeing it as a beautiful journey, a journey of self-awareness and self-improvement.
And we come back to the question of whether we have a problem of will. Our problem is that we don't really know what we want. Unfortunately, no one has taught us how to claim a healthier body and a better life. Nobody has taught us how to live well. Unfortunately, this valuable knowledge is not provided by our education, maybe because it is simply not beneficial to be healthy; not needing medicines, slimming institutes, various complicated diets and food cravings is not profitable. The more we fight against nature, the more and heavier the physical and mental health effects will be. But there is a way, as long as we want to follow it; so let us each explore whether we are willing to respect our nature and wish to change our way of life and thinking...

Sincerely, Elisavet P.

PS: I would like to thank the people who helped me find the right path and gave me the courage and knowledge to walk it. I mainly want to thank them because they believed and still believe in me and support me with patience to find harmony with my nature and regain my lost balance. Mr. Zoumbaneas and Mrs Schina are rare human beings, and I sincerely appreciate you all for conscientiously serving your science, as well as your love and respect for fellow human beings. And this is rare and priceless nowadays.

10th letter

Author's note: Sometimes, trying to motivate people who deal with eating disorders, we recommend writing two letters to their symptom that troubles them. Following is an excellent sample of a young girl who was asked to write a) a letter to bulimia about how she imagined herself, still experiencing bulimia symptoms up to five years later and b) how she imagined herself her and her life without the symptom of bulimia five years later. Let's look at Margarita's letters...

Letter to bulimia

How will I be with bulimia 5 years later.

Dear Bulimia,
Five years ago, I started taking care of my diet more effectively. You didn't like that I was going to leave you... we used to hang out a lot. So, you started biting me like a wild black wolf. You started devouring me and then mending my wounds. You polluted my thinking so that I couldn't think straight. You greedy and insidiously ate away my security and I was in a panic, trying to fill the gaps as fast as I could, the only way I have known how – eating. Mostly with sweets... not coincidentally, right? I think you know what I'm talking about!
Your pressure was so intense that I couldn't resist anymore, and I led myself in your arms again. I gained all the pounds and inches I had lost. You see... the word "lose" in itself creates a void. And I didn't just gain what I had lost. I gained even more to prove to you how loyal I was. Maybe this was how I apologized for attempting to betray our relationship.
Now 5 years later ... I hate you as I've never hated anything in my life before. I hate the part of myself that nourishes you... It hurts to fail to love myself, my thinking, and my body. You deprived me of another 5 years of my life, another five years of oxygen. You made me afraid of a new beginning. Your attacks are very ferocious... so?

Bulimia+Margarita=Lasting Hate to Me
How Scary!

Letter to bulimia

How will I be with bulimia 5 years later.

Dear Bulimia,
Five years ago, I started taking care of my body, as a whole and in a meaningful way. You became determined to destroy me. You used all your tricks. But I had already begun recognising and learning how to manage them.

You sent Sirens to seduce me, and after they had done so, they turned into guilts to drive me mad. But I reconciled with them... we talked things over, I explained to them, and they didn't come back. You became furious! But I don't mind. I found the "straw" with which you were sucking my energy, and I tore it from my veins. You had to see your face when you tried to feed on my energy again, only to realize that it was in vain! You wanted to kill me, but you no longer had access. I had disarmed all your weapons!

Now, five years later, I want to thank you for getting me there. Your war has made me stronger. I developed my thinking, my sensitivity; I went deeper into the path of consciousness. I now live my life being alive...and not by accident! I stopped blocking the flow of energy, the flow of life ... and beautiful things began happening to me, wonderful experiences! Thank you for challenging me so much that I managed to believe in myself. I know that wasn't your goal, but it turned out well for me.

Now that we haven't talked for so long, I wanted to send this letter to you so I can talk to you with love. We spent many years together, and you were close to me in the moments of my most cruel solitude. You also played your part once in my getting through a difficult time! "Thank you. I may one day send you a letter or postcard from new places!

xx

With love,

My Margarita

6.2 Food for Thought

Finishing this book, I would like to present two texts that can really provide food for further thought and discussion...

6.2.1 A Diet Experiment

The first symptoms on human health from prolonged reduced calorie intake have already been reported since the 1950s. Professor Ancel Keys, a student at the University of Minneapolis, published "The Biology of Human Starvation", which was based on a study of 32 healthy and normal weighing men who participated in an effort to reproduce the food intake conditions experienced by civilians and soldiers during World War II in terms of ingested energy from food and food quality. The conditions of the experiment were as follows:

- Their daily calorie intake was decreased from 6,800 to 1,600 calories for 6 months.
- Their diet consisted mainly of carbohydrate, low fat, and low protein through a miniscule amount of meat.
- They joined a daily program of increased physical activity.
- During the six-month study, men developed severe problems like:
- 25% suffered weight loss.
- 40% had a decrease in their metabolic rate.
- 50% had a decrease in cardiac output.
- 20% had a reduction in heart volume.
- They all showed muscular atrophy in the hands and feet that never recovered.
- They all showed symptoms such as a constant feeling of cold in the body, constant fatigue, various mental symptoms such as nervousness, decreased self-esteem, total loss of good mood, and a strong desire for isolation.

All men also developed various negative traits and generally began to be hostile, apathetic, disagreeable, very often irritable, and had severe depression symptoms. Unable to obey the rules, they often went on bulimic episodes and vomiting accompanied by feelings of guilt. Some of them had to be hospitalized in a psychiatric clinic. At the end of the diet, all men gained more than 10% weight compared to the beginning of the experiment, prior to the six-month-long procedure. This was mainly in fat, which was stored in such a way that gave them a relaxed and round appearance in contrast to the muscular and vigorous body shape they had before the study began.

6.2.2 The Secret to Happiness

Many people believe that by slimming, they will also find happiness. But happiness is a multifactorial condition. People often spend much of their time chasing after what they think will give them the coveted happiness. Still, when they finally mee their goal, it doesn't seem to change much in them. The reason? Let this article published in the scientific journal *New Scientist* reveals its secrets.

Which is the secret to happiness? Wealth, beauty, friends, a good marriage or maybe faith? None of this... The most important thing is to inherit the right genes, according to a new study.

The study was compiled by the scientific journal *New Scientist,* which rated (on a scales of 0 - 5) the ten factors that have been proven to be related to human happiness. According to findings, the genetic predisposition to happiness is more important to happiness than a successful marriage, loyal friends, wealth, or religious faith. The truth is that how happy those people feel is partially due to their experience. The other half depends on natural happiness, defined 90% by genes, as studies in twins have shown. This means that people are naturally happy or unhappy. Two people with different genetic susceptibility and other experiences will react differently, leaving one feeling satisfied and the other sad.

6.2.3 The Interviews

The study of *New Scientist* - based on interviews with psychologists and behavioural experts - rates genes 5 out of 5 with scores higher than any other factor. According to Dr. David Laiken, a psychologist at the University of Minnesota, the importance of genes has been proven by numerous studies. One of them took place among 4,000 adult twins who were born in Minnesota, between 1936 and 1955. The second secret to happiness is a successful marriage, rated 3 out of 5. The value of marriage has been demonstrated, among other things, by an international study, that showed that married people are happier than bachelors. Of course, wedding happiness is at its peak a year before the wedding until a year after it. Still, as it diminishes with time, it has a permanent positive effect - as long as it does not corrode along the way. The third scientific key to happiness identified by *New Scientist* is the acquisition and retention of loyal friends. A study by the University of Illinois showed that Calcutta's slum dwellers are just as happy as the city's middle-income students. The close friendship ties, according to the researchers. Friendship was rated 2.5 out of 5 on the *New scientist* scales.

The Times, 2003

6.2.4 The List of Happiness

Agent	Rating out (out of 5)
Genetic predisposition	5
Successful marriage	3
Loyal friends	2,5
Low expectations	2
Giving to others	1,5
Faith	1,5
Appearance	1
Wealth	0,5
Good old age	0,5
Intelligence	0

New Scientist

6.3 Bibliography

Dingemans A. E., et al., Binge eating disorder: a review. International Journal of Obesity, 2002.

Donnellan Craig, Eating Disorders, Vol. 127.

Fairburn Christofer and Wilson Terence, Eating Disorders and Obesity.

Geary Amanda, The Food and Mood Handbook.

Gilbert Sarah, Counselling for Eating Disorders.

Goleman Daniel, The Emotional Intelligence.

Huther Gerald, Manual of the Human Brain.

Jade Deanne, Training Manuals, www.eating-disorders.org.uk

www.Diatrofi.gr

Training of Eating Disorders, www.keadd.gr

6.4 Websites

www.diatrofi.gr
www.eating-disorders.org.uk
www.eating-disorders.com
www.keadd.gr
www.nationaleatingdisorders.org

Reader's Feedback

- An outstanding effort, well worth rewarding and will undoubtedly be read... scientific concepts given in a simple and comprehensive way for the average everyday person… to process our general behaviour and not just the part of nutrition, which is a trigger for improvement ... as humans ...
- It is a book written with sensitivity, that reveals the author's training and experience on the subject as well as his genuine interest in the person behind the problem. It includes useful nutritional tips and habits you can adopt to get the desired result, making it clear that no magic recipes exist. I would say that the examples cited above work encouragingly. It is essential that, through analysis, they show that the "battle" for a "slimmer" self is ultimately part of everyone's quest for self-awareness.
- It is an excellent book, written in a comprehensive manner by a man with immense experience on the subject, structured to be understood by everyone, even those who do not possess specialized knowledge. The writer's reporting of facts helps the average reader better understand nutritional concepts. This book has the most psychological and emotional approach to bulimic episodes I've read. The Nutrition Intelligence Index is a weapon for every person that, if used properly, can help its holder remain healthy, free of unnecessary weight, and maintain high wellness levels. I was thrilled to read it and would highly recommend it to everyone.
- Growing up in a traditional family in which the Mediterranean diet was dominant, I often wondered whether my diet was right. What I have found from time to time is that everyone

has their own opinion on the subject. Reading your book everything became clearer in my mind. The simple and straightforward way it develops serious and crucial issues helps the reader understand what is ultimately true. Finishing this book, I put some previously unassorted thoughts in order. I am now convinced of what the right diet is. It is worth noting that even if we go astray, we should not give up our goal: healthy and proper nutrition. As you say, a new day starts, and we have to continue from where we left off. Maybe ignorance... is what makes us fat?

- Nutritional Intelligence and beyond

  Good evening, Mr Zoumbaneas,

  The truth is, I expected your book to be one of the same, similar to all the American self-improvement books that treat every issue in a similar fashion ... Thankfully it isn't.

  I want to congratulate you, not because you have made some remarkable discovery, but because you really know what we mean when talking about a "binge-eating episode" and present it with the proper importance. Most people (even dietitians) think that we like to eat a lot and treat us like children who have been disobedient and should be punished for it (as if self-punishment is not enough).

  I was also amazed at the logic of 'knowledge is power' and your attempt to teach people to feed themselves, instead of feeding them. Unfortunately, in the age of commercialization, most people try to sell you their "fish", but rarely do they tell you where and how they fished them.

  Let me also tell you that your writing way is totally comprehensive, even for a child, which is very important, especially in describing the various nutrient absorption mechanisms. I will tell you the things I did not like once I have read it a second time, because during the first reading I found nothing.

  I have to admit that you have put me in the game, Mr. Zoumbaneas because now I know how it is played in my body and mind.

- NUTRITIONAL INTELLIGENCE FOR ALL, AND FOR US !!!

  Everyone congratulates you on this book, and I am sincerely

thrilled about it!!! I will talk about the power of our work, that unconscionable people have taken advantage of to fill their pockets, without considering human pain and the unpleasant consequences this can have on their patient. Is it worth sacrificing everything for money and fame? Is our work only about the number of diets we will create, what commission we will get and what will be the bonus that we can achieve? Who is considered a SUCCESSFUL DIETITIAN? The patients themselves will make us successful and they will also reject us, so, let us put a little more effort in dealing with them. I want to say that you are a SUCCESSFUL person, not because you wrote a book but because you recorded many years of work in a book for us and your job is worth more!!! NUTRITIONAL INTELLIGENCE: A COURSE BOOK FOR EVERYONE.

Ioanna B., Nutritionist

- Mr Zoumbaneas, taking the courage to contact you, I would like to congratulate you on the book Nutritional Intelligence.

  Even though I am studying to become a nutritionist and have never had a weight problem, it is amazing how quickly different influences managed to throw me into the world of eating disorders and deep depression. I have been struggling for a year now, trying to get away from the obsessions that have been consuming me every day! I thought I wouldn't be able to feel normal again. I'm still scared that all this will come back and drag me down again. Binge eating, vomiting, pills, over-eating. They are the black hole of my life. In 2.5 months, I gained 15 kilos and became self-destructive! I still don't remember the day I started caring for myself again and getting away from it all. Before I got into the binge eating episodes (after the binge eating episodes) I read your book, applied the diet and I was surprised when I got on the weighing scales and had lost the weight I wanted to, eating properly. Due to health and medication problems and an unconscionable dietitian, who exhausted me on a nutritional level, as she was clueless, I began gaining weight and the situation escalated from there! Having escaped from all this, I know what I went through will be a valuable life lesson, and your book will be a crucial guide in my later career in Nutrition. I even recommended it to the dietitian I mentioned above to save others from what I went through, though I don't have high hopes. Keep up the good work because in a world of charlatans and supposed "scientists", we need the right standards to support our course with confidence, us, the next generation! Thanks for your time, and I hope one day I will become an equally good nutritionist!

6.5 Key Takeaways

1. **Embrace self-awareness:**
   - Recognize the connection between your emotions and eating habits.
   - Understanding the reason behind your food choices can help you regain control.
2. **Small steps lead to big changes:**
   - Start with manageable adjustments to your diet and lifestyle rather than aiming for drastic changes.
   - Consistency is more important than perfection.
3. **Stress and eating are linked:**
   - Learn how stress affects your hunger and cravings.
   - Practice techniques like mindfulness or deep breathing to manage stress without turning to food.
4. **Food is nourishment, not a coping mechanism:**
   - Shift your mindset to see food as fuel for your body and mind, rather than a way to deal with emotions.
   - Balanced meals can boost your energy and mood.
5. **The role of routine:**
   - Establish regular eating patterns to help your body maintain stability.
   - Prioritize nutritious foods to support your overall well-being.
6. **You are not alone:**
   - Seeking guidance from professionals or sharing your experiences with others within the context of a therapeutic group can make a huge difference.
   - Support systems can empower you to overcome challenges.

7. **Celebrate progress, not perfection:**
   - Acknowledge and appreciate the effort you put into improving your relationship with food.
   - Every small success is a step toward long-term health and happiness.

Chapter 7

Understanding the Voice of Disorder

The best patient is the one who needs his/her therapist to confirm how good they are...

7.1 Frequently Asked Questions from the Environment of Those Struggling with Eating Disorders

Excerpt from NEDAParentToolkit edited by Research Associates from the Centre for Education and Treatment of Eating Disorders

Eating Disorders can be confusing even for health professionals who have been involved in treating them for years. This is partly because they are surrounded by numerous myths and misconceptions. It may be difficult for some people to properly diagnose an eating disorder. This section will help resolve some of the most common misconceptions about eating disorders and those affected by them.

Eating disorders are an option. Is it just enough to tell my beloved to overcome the problem?

Eating disorders (EDS) are complex medical and psychiatric illnesses that patients do not choose to go through, and parents do not cause.

Nutritional Intelligence: The Answer to Bulimia, Overeating, and Obesity
Evangelos Zoumbaneas

ISBN 978-981-5129-74-8 (Hardcover), 978-981-5129-73-1 (Paperback), 978-1-003-65188-8 (eBook)
www.jennystanford.com

In the Diagnostic and Statistical Manual, 5th Edition Diagnostic and Statistical Manual, 5th Edition (DSM-5)] The American Psychiatric Association classifies eating disorders in five different types: anorexia nervosa, bulimia nervosa, obsessive-compulsive binge eating, restrictive eating disorder and no otherwise identified eating disorder. Several decades of genetic research have shown that hereditary and biological factors play an essential role in developing an eating disorder. Eating disorders generally occur along with other mental health conditions, such as depression, anxiety, social phobia or obsessive-compulsive disorder.

Do we all have an eating disorder nowadays?

Although our modern culture is obsessed with food and body weight, and disrupted eating habits are common, clinical manifestations of eating disorders are not as frequent. A 2007 study examined 9,282 English-speaking Americans with various mental disorders, including eating disorders. Results published in Biological Sciences found that during their lifetime, 0.9% of women and 0.3% of men suffered from anorexia nervosa, 1.5% of women and 1.5% of men developed bulimia nervosa, 3.5% women and 2.0% men experienced episodic binge eating. The consequences of eating disorders can be life-threatening, and many people find that stigma due to mental illness (and eating disorders in particular) can prevent early diagnosis and proper treatment.

Are eating disorders an option?

The causes of an eating disorder are complex. According to modern researchers and clinical experts, eating disorders are caused by both genetic and environmental factors. They are "bio-socio-cultural" diseases. One social aspect is the media promotion of the image of a lean body as the 'ideal'. It is an environmental factor associated with increased risk of developing eating disorders. Environmental factors also include various physical ailments, teasing, and bullying during childhood and other stressful life situations. Historical evidence reveals that some of the first documented cases of eating disorders were associated with religious fasting. Also, eating disorders are usually inherited in families. There is a biological predisposition that makes individuals more vulnerable to developing an eating disorder.

I want to understand what I did to cause my child to have an eating disorder.

Organizations worldwide, including the Academy for Eating Disorders of the American Psychiatric Association and NEDA have published guidelines that show that parents do not cause eating disorders. Parents, especially mothers, were traditionally blamed for children's eating disorders. Still, more recent research suggests that these disorders have a strong biological root. They develop differently in each affected individual; there is no single set of rules that guarantees that, if observed by parents, the development of an eating disorder can be prevented. However, there are some things that everyone in their family can do to help create an environment that promotes recovery from the disorder. Psychologists have significantly impacted the recovery speed for children and adolescents when parents are involved in the treatment process.

If the eating disorder is not diagnosed early, can it develop into a big problem we will have to deal with?

Eating disorders have the highest mortality rate than any other mental illness. Up to 20% of people with chronic anorexia nervosa will die from the disease. Studies on anorexia, bulimia and Unspecified Feeding or Eating Disorder (UFED) show that all eating disorders have similarly elevated mortality rates. In addition to medical complications from excessive eating, purging methods, starvation and overexercising, suicide is prevalent in people with eating disorders. Also, people suffering from eating disorders can experience severe consequences in their quality of life.

Is anorexia the only serious eating disorder?

When researchers looked at the death rates in people with any diagnosis of eating disorders treated as outpatients, they found that bulimia and undetermined eating disorders (UFED now OSFED) had similarly high mortality rates, similar to those of anorexia nervosa. During the study, about 1 of 20 people with eating disorders lost their lives because of their illness. Patients who abuse laxatives or diuretics or cause vomiting are at a significantly higher risk of sudden death from heart attacks due to electrolyte imbalances.

Excessive exercise can also increase the risk of death in people with eating disorders, increasing physical stress levels.

Since I do not see my child having an eating disorder behaviour, do I have to worry?

Many people with eating disorders are forced to hide the symptoms of their illness, either because of shame or because they are afraid that someone will stop them. For the people close to the person struggling with the disorder, it is not uncommon to be surprised by how severe and corrosive eating disorder behaviours are after it is diagnosed. If you know a loved one who is suffering from an eating disorder, it is essential to express your concern with sympathy and compassion and encourage the person to seek help.

If my child is not ready to recover from his/her eating disorder, is there anything I can do until they get to that point?

Some people with eating disorders have difficulty identifying their illness or assessing the severity of their condition. On the other hand, some patients may desperately want to stop their disordered behaviour, but they are afraid. While the sufferer's expression of and willingness to recover from the disorder can be a positive sign, treatment does not have to wait until your loved ones are ready. If they are under the age of 18, or otherwise, it is imperative that treatment must start as soon as possible - once you are aware of the problem. Early intervention is associated with significantly higher recovery rates. If the sufferer is an adult, family and friends should continue to express their concerns about the negative impact of eating disorders on their loved one's life and encourage them to seek help from a specialist.

As a parent, are there things I can do to help my child recover from eating disorder?

Although research continues "until proven otherwise," parental involvement in the treatment of a child's eating disorder can increase the chances of recovery. Some types of treatment, such as family therapy, provide that parents temporarily take full control of the child's diet and monitor for any purging procedures until a healthy weight is achieved and healthy eating habits are re-established. Other loved ones can continue to support the eating disorder patient, helping to reduce eating stress and reminding them that it is just a disease. Even if you decide that family therapy does not suit your family, there are still many ways you can participate in the treatment of your child or loved one.

Will my family member who suffers not recover until the cause of his/her eating disorder is discovered?

While some may find a reason or cause that they believe was the ground for their eating disorder, most people suffering from such diseases can't account for their existence. There is no evidence that discovering the cause of an eating disorder is associated with recovering from it. Regardless of the reason why someone may have developed an eating disorder, usually the priority of treatment is to restore normal nutrition and body weight.

If my loved one insists that they are fine, should I believe them?

Problems with self-awareness are one of the main features of eating disorders. Therefore, your loved one may not have the self-awareness needed to recognize the problem caused by the disorder. The sufferer may genuinely believe that he is well until he reaches a marginal and life-threatening point. Others may deny having an eating disorder even when they feel sick because they are afraid of treatment. Regardless of the reason, it is essential that we insist on the need for supervision by a mental health professional trained in eating disorders and regular medical monitoring by a physician experienced in this field.

Isn't having strict dietary rules or applying different types of diet-style dietary patterns a problem?

It seems that the implementation of a "strict" diet can actually trigger an eating disorder. Even if the symptoms do not fully meet the criteria for a clinical diagnosis of an eating disorder, disordered eating habits can have serious health consequences, such as anaemia and osteopenia. People with a severe eating disorder can benefit from early intervention and treatment to address their anxieties before the condition develops into an eating disorder. Chronic dieting has been associated with the subsequent development of an eating disorder; therefore, immediate response to such issues may prevent its development.

If someone is not too thin, does it mean that they are not suffering from some kind of eating disorder?

Most people suffering from an eating disorder are not underweight. Although most sufferers are portrayed by the media as extremely thin, an eating disorder cannot be determined solely by the individual's appearance. These perceptions can perpetuate the problem and cause discomfort to people with eating disorders. They may find that they are not "sick enough" or "well enough", depending on the disorder, to require treatment. You also cannot determine if a person has a binge eating disorder based solely on their weight. It is important to remember that just because the sufferer is no longer scrawny or has lost weight in treating a binge eating disorder does not mean that he has recovered completely. A person can experience a severe form of eating disorder, whatever his/her weight.

Is the main symptom of eating disorder that I have to worry about losing weight?

Although anorexia nervosa and other restrictive eating disorders are characterized by weight loss, many people with eating disorders do not lose weight or may even gain weight due to their disorder.

Are eating disorders focused only on eating?

People with eating disorders generally have an unhealthy attitude towards food and weight. Still, the symptoms of an eating disorder can extend to issues far beyond nutrition. Many scientific studies have shown a correlation between eating disorders, perfectionism, and obsessive-compulsive/compulsive behaviours, leading to an obsession with grades, athletic performance, etc. Many sufferers report that eating disorder behaviours initially helped them reduce their levels of depression and anxiety; but, as the disorder progresses, malnutrition caused by eating disorders can eventually increase these levels and affect all aspects of life.

My child or my partner no longer claims feeling fat. Could they still have an eating disorder?

Absolutely. Body image disorder perceived by the sufferer is prevalent in eating disorders, but it is far from universal. Clinical reports show that young children are less likely to have body image disorder and the majority of adolescents and adults do not report this symptom.

Given that eating disorders are linked to heredity, is it correct to assume that my child or partner has little hope of recovery?

It is important to remember that heredity is not destiny. There is always hope for recovery. Although hereditary factors play a significant role in the onset of eating disorders, they are not the only cause. Predisposition for disordered eating behaviour may resurface in times of stress. Still, there are many useful techniques with which people with eating disorders can learn to manage their emotions appropriately and avoid returning to disturbing behaviours.

I have a son. Do I have to worry about eating given that eating disorders mainly affect women?

Eating disorders can affect anyone, regardless of gender or origin. Although they are more common in women, researchers and clinicians find that more and more men are seeking help for such issues. A 2007 study by the Centre for Disease Control and Prevention found that up to one-third of all people with eating disorders are men. It is unclear whether there is a real increase of such disorders in men or whether more male sufferers are now seeking treatment, or if more men are being diagnosed. Since doctors do not believe that eating disorders affect men, in general, their symptoms become more severe before they are diagnosed. There may be subtle differences in thoughts about food consumption and disordered behaviour in men, so they are more likely to focus on increasing muscle mass than losing weight. They are also more likely to purge through exercise and steroid abuse than women. Although homosexual, bisexual, and transgender (men) are more likely to develop eating disorders than their heterosexual counterparts, the overwhelming majority of men with eating disorders are heterosexuals.

Is my child too young to develop an eating disorder?

Eating disorders can develop or recur at any age. Eating disorder experts report an increase in eating disorders among children, even at the age of five or six. Many people suffering from eating disorders report that their unhealthy thoughts and behaviours started much earlier than one might imagine, sometimes even in their early teens. Selective eating is common in young children but does not necessarily prove the existence of an eating disorder. Although most report the development of an eating disorder during their adolescence and early adulthood, some patients are diagnosed at an earlier age. It is unclear whether there is an increase in eating disorders at younger generations or whether increased awareness of eating disorders has led to the improvement of their identification and diagnosis in young children.

Now that my child or my partner is no longer a teenager, do I need to worry about an eating disorder?

People can suffer from an eating disorder regardless of their age. Literature survey has highlighted a subset of people with eating disorders who appear to have spontaneously recovered from their illness without treatment. However, many people who suffer from such disorders and have been eating in a disordered manner since adolescence, continue to suffer during adulthood unless they receive proper treatment. Middle-aged men and women as well as older people are often treated for eating disorders due to either relapsing or their illness persisting since their adolescence or adulthood, or the emergence of a new eating disorder.

Is it possible that I should not worry about my child or my partner? After all, anyone can eat too much ice cream sometimes...

Binge eating disorder affects only 3.5% of women, 2% of men, and up to 1.6% of adolescents. It is not the same thing as occasionally eating more than what is necessary. Those suffering from binge eating disorder are involved in a cycle of recurrent binge eating episodes - at least once a week for more than three months - in which they consume significantly more food in a short time than most people might. The frequency and severity of the disorder have significant and adverse effects on one's life, with many suffering from coexisting diseases such as depression and anxiety disorder.

My child and/or my partner have bulimia. So, there is no chance of developing another type of eating disorder.

Many patients with eating disorders will suffer from more than one eating disorder before they finally recover. About half of the people who suffer anorexia will develop bulimia. Some people show signs of anorexia and bulimia simultaneously, with frequent episodes of over-eating, and may also apply purging techniques despite having low weight (this condition is clinically classified as bulimia/purging anorexia). Still, some patients may switch from one diagnosis to another, a process also known as crossover diagnosis. All of this can have life-threatening consequences.

Does purging only mean vomiting?

Purging involves any method of "removing" food from the body before it is fully digested. Often, the individual is driven to purging to compensate for what he considers to be excessive intake of food. Self-inflicted vomiting is one of the most common methods one can use, but not the only one. Laxatives and enema may also be used, as well as non-purging compensatory behaviours, such as misuse of insulin, fasting, excessive exercise, and more. More than one purging method may also be used. Each method involves its own risks, but all of them involve potentially life-threatening electrolyte imbalances.

Once my child, who suffers from anorexia, gains weight, will he or she be fine?

Restoring weight and the state of nutrition is just the first step in recovering from anorexia. Once the sufferer of anorexia nervosa returns to a weight which is healthy for him or her, he or she can participate more fully and substantially in psychotherapy. Significant psychological work must be done so that one can manage difficult emotions without resorting to anorexic behaviours. Weight loss alone does not mean that the disorder has been cured.

Seeking treatment for loved one with eating disorder.

According to the Panhellenic Research on Eating Disorders conducted by CETED in collaboration with the European University of Cyprus in 2018, a large percentage of patients - over 50% - with small or more serious weight problems, have some type of eating disorder. If this is not diagnosed as soon as possible and is simply treated as yet another common case, the patient will either discontinue any form of treatment or relapse within the next two months. People suffering from any form of eating disorder need special treatment and specialized healing skills to remain in any treatment scheme until the end of their treatment. Getting the right diagnosis of eating disorder from an experienced health professional is just the first step towards recovery.

Many eating disorder sufferers can be treated as outpatients, so it is essential for any health practitioner - dietitian to have experience in handling eating disorders. A primary care physician, such as a paediatrician, physician, or family doctor, may refer the patient to another therapist, e.g., a dietitian experienced in the treatment of eating disorders, and other specialties e.g., a psychologist and/or a physical education teacher. Experience has shown that treating eating disorders with a collaborating treatment team to address the many aspects of an eating disorder is the optimal approach. Treatment groups usually include the following types of specialists:

- Doctor (primary care physician, paediatrician, cardiologist, etc.)
- Psychologist
- Dietitian
- Psychiatrist
- Physical education teacher

7.2 The Need for Specialised Knowledge and Therapeutic Tools

The knowledge and skills acquired by each health professional through the program Master Practitioner on Eating Disorders, provided exclusively by the Centre for Education and Treatment of Eating Disorders, will distinguish the skilled therapist who will be able to provide every therapeutic approach, thus creating a feeling of constant and permanent interaction with his patient.

Eating disorders and emotional eating disorders occur not only when patients seek help with specific nutritional issues, but also through other emotional and physical disorders. The ability to help others regain a healthy relationship with food, and therefore themselves, is a vital tool for health professionals.

The course combines many therapeutic methods. Firstly, based on cognitive-behavioural therapy. The educational material is presented in the form of lectures, small group exercises, role exercises, diagnostic exercises, and exercises in acquiring specific skills.

7.3 Master Practitioner in Eating Disorders & Obesity Course

The training course covers a total of 120 hours. It takes place during 8 weekends in Athens and Thessaloniki by physical or online attendance, as well as watching "on demand" videos of the recorded lessons for up to 3 working days after the end of every instructional weekend.

Seek recorded video clips and information on the official website www.keadd.gr by the Centre for Education and Treatment of Eating Disorders.

7.4 Key Takeaways

1. Understand your triggers:
    - Identify emotional or situational triggers that influence your eating habits.
    - Awareness is the first step to breaking the cycle of emotional eating.
2. **Emotional hunger vs. physical hunger:**
    - Learn to differentiate between emotional eating and eating for nourishment.
    - Physical hunger comes gradually, while emotional hunger often feels sudden and urgent.

3. **Develop healthier coping mechanisms:**
   - Replace food as a coping tool with activities like journaling, walking, or talking to a friend.
   - Stress management techniques, such as mindfulness or meditation, can also help.
4. **Practice self-compassion:**
   - Avoid criticizing yourself for momentary events of emotional eating. Everyone occasionally succumbs to such urges.
   - Focus on progress, not perfection, as you build healthier habits.
5. **Rebuild your relationship with food:**
   - View food as a source of nourishment and enjoyment, not as a reward or punishment.
   - Create balanced meals that satisfy both your body and mind.
6. **Set realistic goals:**
   - Break your goals into small, achievable steps that feel manageable.
   - Celebrate every positive change, no matter how small it seems.
7. **Reach out for support:**
   - You don't have to do it alone. Seek professional help to guide you through your journey, but do not forget the support of your friends, and family.
   - Support networks can keep you motivated and accountable.

Chapter 8

The Importance of Proper Diagnosis of the Disorder

I always prefer curing people to treating metrics...

8.1 What Do the First Results of Research on Eating Disorders in Greece Reveal

The Centre for Education and Treatment of Eating Disorders, headed by Mr. Evangelos Zoumbaneas, in collaboration with the European University of Cyprus, conducted a panhellenic-scales research, designed and organized by the Professor of Education on Eating Disorders, Vassileios E. Katsilas, with the participation of 25 external collaborators and under scientific supervision for the proper and scientifically sound realization of Assistant Professor Panagiotis Petrou.

The study's design was based on the internationally accredited Eating Disorders Detection Protocol taught in CETED in combination with behavioural questions and demographic characteristics for new clients of a nutritionist by a trained dietitian-nutritionist.

The study sample was 625 people and consisted of people from every geographical region of Greece.

The results of the survey are enlightening. Figure 8.1 shows an analysis of some of the most important findings:

Nutritional Intelligence: The Answer to Bulimia, Overeating, and Obesity
Evangelos Zoumbaneas

ISBN 978-981-5129-74-8 (Hardcover), 978-981-5129-73-1 (Paperback), 978-1-003-65188-8 (eBook)
www.jennystanford.com

As we can see in the graph above, it appears that about 65% of people who visit the office of a dietitian-nutritionist have lost and regained more than 9% during their lives through diet at least once (see the table below a more detailed analysis of the results). This result presents a risk for a possible biochemical imbalance as we do not know the nature of the chosen diet and followed by each participant (e.g., ketogenic diet, diuretics, slimming pills, laxatives, etc.), nor if it was followed with a scientifically acceptable manner (with the help of a certified dietitian-nutritionist). We can also conclude that, in addition to physical biochemistry, repeated weight loss and weight gain adversely affect one's mental health.

Does the number on the weighing scales affect your mood and the way you see yourself throughout the day (Figure 8.1)?

Have you lost and regained > 9 kg in your life through a Diet?

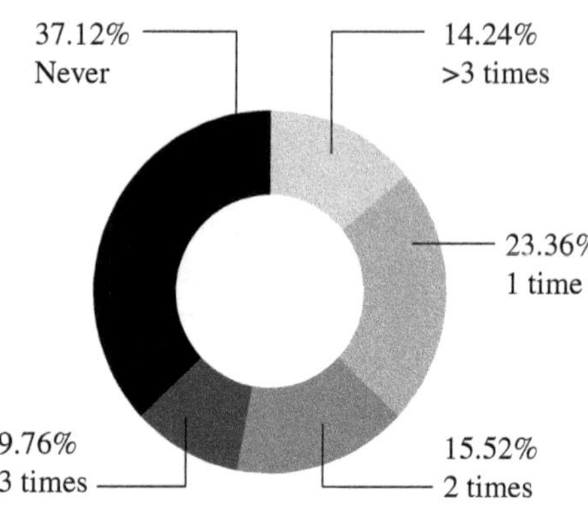

Figure 8.1

In Figure 8.2, we can see that one's overall mental health throughout the day is simply influenced by a number, affecting the mood and the way one sees oneself throughout the day.

The weighing scales is one of the most widespread and perhaps most established measuring systems for a person's progress while losing excessive weight. It is essential for any professional dietitian not to use a weighing scale as a means of assessment and to be trained in other assessment methods that encourage and enhance the patient's overall diet.

Then we see that the percentage of people who weigh themselves regularly during a week and month is very high, which, as we have seen above, has a huge impact on their mental health (Figure 8.3).

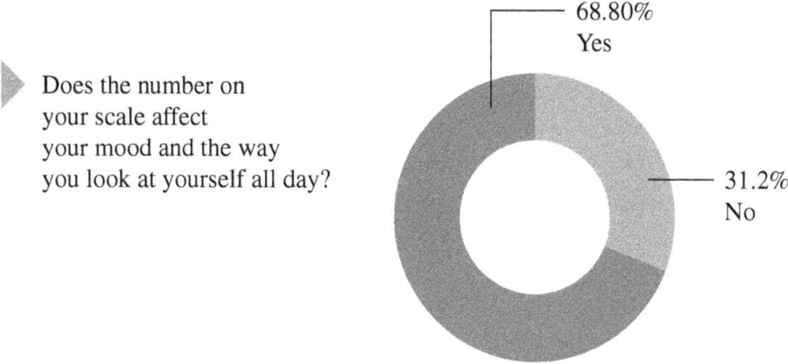

Figure 8.2

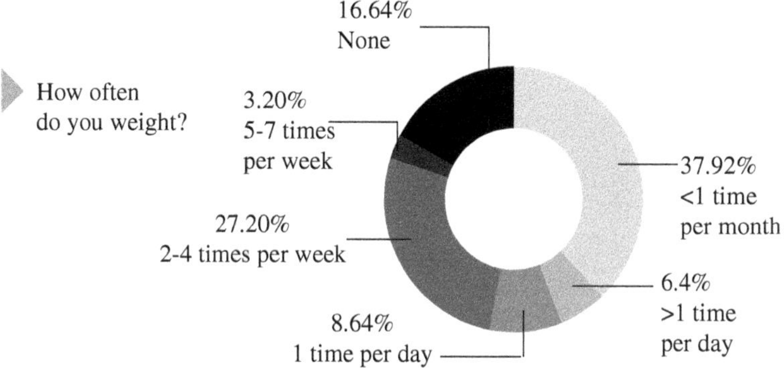

Figure 8.3

The graph in Figure 8.4 shows that more than half of those who visit a professional dietitian's-nutritionist's office think they are overweight even though others say they are not. One of the main characteristics of an eating disorder is that the person has a misconception about his / her body image, which is evident in the graph above. Client body image modification and enhancement techniques are important tools for the progress and duration of the client's treatment.

The prevalence of eating disorders among clients of the nutritionists participating in the study is of particular interest (Figure 8.5). One of the most important findings is that 1 in 4 people (25%) who come to a dietitian's office suffer from an eating disorder. This result is based on the stricter specifications because if we review cases of people who are just approaching the specifications of the evaluation model indicating someone having an eating disorder, the result is much greater. This is also the main reason why 25% of each dietitian's clients stop their effort in less than two months, or at the first indication that the result on the weighing scales does not meet their expectations (which are usually overly optimistic).

Do you feel that you are overweight even though others tell you that you are not?

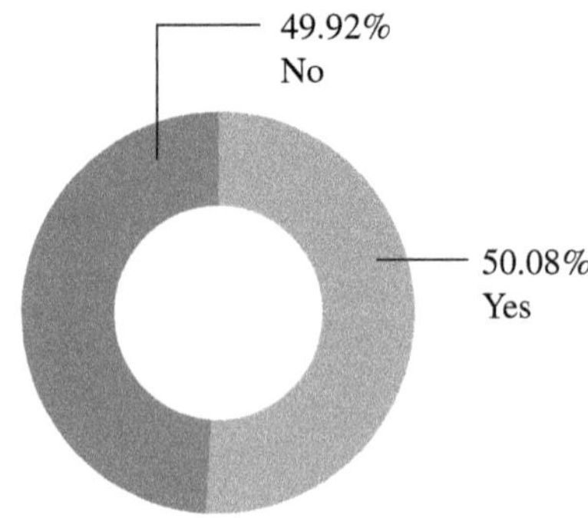

Figure 8.4

Percentage of an eating disorder incident

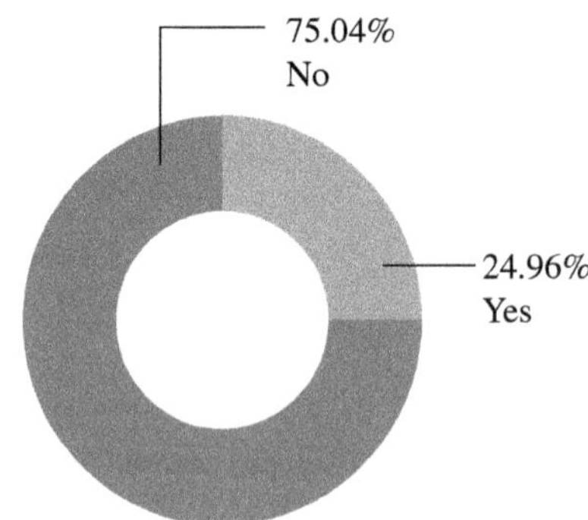

Figure 8.5

Eighteen percent of people have some kind of eating disorder and are unaware of it (Figure 8.6).

Nearly 1 in 5 clients are unaware that they are suffering from an eating disorder; a lack of knowledge of the proper diagnosis of the disease will soon be the main reason for the client to stop going to the dietitian and will then look for another, until they recognize the symptoms of the disorder and apply appropriate therapeutic tools and techniques to cure the symptoms of the disease.

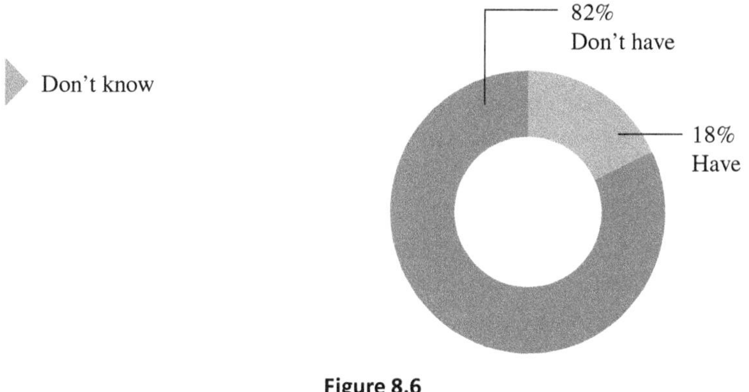

Figure 8.6

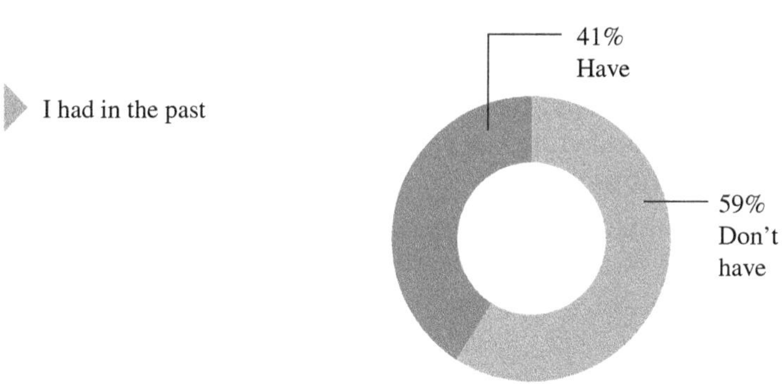

Figure 8.7

Forty one percent of those who responded that they had an eating disorder in the past still suffer from such a disorder (Figure 8.7). Many of them have changed many dietitians and often followed too extreme and rigorous diet plans until they came to an experienced professional dietitian, like those of the CETED team, who recognized the eating disorder symptoms and used all the appropriate tools to restore the customer's balance between food and emotional eating.

Simply put, this research has shown that if the nutritionist is not trained to detect and able to cope with any eating disorder, he will lose at least 1/4 of his clientele or drag them even deeper into their eating disorder...

8.2 Key Takeaways

1. **The Importance of Proper Diagnosis**:
    - Proper diagnosis of eating disorders is the cornerstone of effective treatment.
    - Misdiagnoses or overlooking symptoms can lead to worsening of symptoms and patients losing trust in professionals.
2. **Role of Nutritionists**:
    - Nutritionists must recognize the signs of eating disorders to provide targeted therapeutic approaches.
    - Training in this field is essential for preventing patients from being mismanaged or referred elsewhere.
3. **Impact of Eating Disorders**:
    - Eating disorders impact both physical and emotional well-being, often leading to cycles of guilt and frustration if untreated.
    - Addressing these disorders requires a compassionate and informed approach.
4. **Statistical Insights**:
    - A significant proportion of people who have had an eating disorder continue to struggle without proper intervention.
    - Research indicates the need for specialized, continuous care.
5. **Therapeutic Relationships**:
    - Building trust with patients is key to their progress.
    - Effective communication and empathy are essential for understanding the underlying issues behind an individual's eating patterns.
6. **Holistic Approach**:
    - Treatment should encompass emotional, psychological, and nutritional dimensions.
    - Empower patients to manage their condition by fostering self-awareness and resilience.

Chapter 9

Conversations on Eating Disorders

Excerpts from the author's interviews in the Greek press

9.1 Excerpts from the Author's Interviews in the Greek Press

9.1.1 Interview for *ELLE* Magazine by Journalist Georgia Karkani, October 2014

In your opinion, is the term 'food addiction' correct? Is there a risk that we may become addicted to food, or at least to certain ingredients such as sugar, in the sense that this might happen like, for example, with drugs? If so, what are the 'addictive' ingredients?

Across the board, the terms "food addiction" & "eating addiction" describe a disorder that has not yet been fully elucidated. The former, describes the disorder of a person's addiction to a certain food or food ingredients, while the latter is used to denote an addiction to the process of eating in general. However, it has not yet been scientifically documented that there is an addiction to food ingredients, such as sugar, similar to that caused by alcohol or

Nutritional Intelligence: The Answer to Bulimia, Overeating, and Obesity
Evangelos Zoumbaneas

ISBN 978-981-5129-74-8 (Hardcover), 978-981-5129-73-1 (Paperback), 978-1-003-65188-8 (eBook)
www.jennystanford.com

nicotine. However, there is an addiction to the process of eating e.g., the opening of the chocolate box, how the person eats it and possibly the environment around it at that time. Normal weighing individuals may also be addicted to food, while obese individuals may have a healthy relationship with food. For survival reasons, the human brain is stimulated when we eat foods high in sugar or fat.

However, it is difficult for us to imagine someone returning home tired from a difficult day, opening the fridge and devouring fruits and vegetables. Still, if there was nothing but fruit in the fridge and he could eat nothing else, he might. After all, what he really wants is to satisfy his fatigue through food, but he would almost certainly stop short of eating 1 kg of cabbage but easily double this if it was ice-cream he was having. So, we understand the difference, and it seems that food addiction is more common, but food addiction is the cause. Devouring large quantities of food, regardless of kind, is more strongly associated with eating disorders, such as bulimia nervosa or orthorexia. Most of us can turn our attention to foods that make us feel well. Usually these foods contain many carbohydrates, sugar and white flour, and commonly calorie-rich foods without many nutrients. This happens because from a very young age, even as infants, we combine e.g., the sweet taste of milk, which relieves us, with care, a loving embrace, even motherly love, thus creating powerful memories or "neuronal synapses" that multiply over the years. For example, at a celebration gathering, the cheerful feelings we experience, and the warm atmosphere are combined with plenty of food, usually rich in calories (chips, soufflés, pizzas, etc.), sweets (e.g., birthday cake), and alcohol. This often leads us to seeking these tastes when we feel sad or tired in order to feel better.

Beyond the psychological part, there is also a physiological aspect that drives us to overeating and addiction. When the body feels hungry, it craves nutrients. We are destined to eat unprocessed, nutrient-rich foods to nourish our cells. Despite the social dimension of food and today's huge level of food processing from the field to our plate, the essence of food is primarily to satisfy the basic survival needs of the body, take in all the ingredients necessary for it to grow and repair the damages done to it and then, achieve mental or social satisfaction. So, when we continuously consume processed foods, our brain gets confused. It doesn't receive enough nutrients and drives us to eat more and more until it meets its micronutrient needs for vitamins, minerals, trace minerals, etc., no matter if the indicated caloric intake from carbohydrates and fats, has far been surpassed.

Usually, addictive foods are high in carbohydrates and fat; less often, one can be addicted to protein-rich foods that cause satiety faster. So, if we don't fill our stomachs or if we don't say STOP, because we are worried that our weight will increase, we could easily empty a whole family-sized ice cream, a family-sized bag of crisps, a jar of praline, etc., instead of eating a whole watermelon, a jar of honey or a boar. This is an addiction; that is why the human brain is somehow addicted to processed foods and so it is thought that e.g., sugar or white flour, or processed salt, which are of no nutritional value and are the first ingredients we read on the labels of all processed foods, cause addiction. Studies from the University of Michigan even estimate that 5 to 10% of the general population is addicted to some kind of food. At the same time, this percentage is higher in obese individuals and those dealing with a binge-eating disorder.

If you agree that there is an addiction to food, how does it relate to other eating disorders such as bulimia, and how should it be treated?

Eating addiction is very similar to alcohol addiction also in how the addict tries to keep his addiction under control. It is associated with eating disorders more like bulimia or binge eating disorder. In anorexia, people are, in some ways, "addicted" even to foods that most people can't get addicted to, for example, rice cookers, lettuce, carrots, 0% fat ice cream, but also foods high in calories and sugar, such as chocolate, ice cream or pizza, which have been included in their rigid schedule, with a strict measure and religious ritual related to their consumption. Often, exhaustive exercise has preceded the meal, or will follow it, or even attempts to purge it in other ways will take place. This addiction also applies to people who feel that they are on a diet. Their daily diet consists of untasteful or psychologically unsatisfactory foods, and habitually consuming "addictive foods," which they even consider "banned," is much more likely and more powerful. There are also strong rules governing their diet e.g., they don't eat anything after 8 pm or eat chocolate only on Sunday. But when such a person starts consuming the first bite of the food he is addicted to, as with alcohol, the addiction is so strong that he cannot stop until he eats as much of that food is available to him. In bulimia, when one type of food is over, the person switches to another and often alters between salty and sweet foods and eventually somehow purging it, while in addiction he usually stops eating as soon as the food causing the reaction is over. In both cases there can be remorse for a number of reasons: in bulimia mainly for fear of weight gain, but also that due to health concerns, being sinful, addicted, ethically condemned etc. This creates a vicious circle, and the addiction becomes impossible to break. The first step in dealing with this is to stop believing that food is forbidden, wrong, sinful, etc. and know that it may be consumed at any time, so that the individual can slowly be satisfied with less. The second step - but taken simultaneously with the first - would be to introduce new, more nutritious, tasty alternatives that satisfy, satiate and leave no room for non-nutritious choices. I think it's wrong for someone to abruptly stop consuming one type of food without having found alternative foods that please and satiate, otherwise the person will sooner or later return to it with greater intensity, unless there is a health problem e.g., diabetes or hypertension. This process is a long one; the individual should be supported by their environment and a specialist who will undertake their proper nutritional retraining.

Regarding our country, from your experience, how has Modern Greece's consumer culture evolved in recent years? Are you looking at, for example, the shift to healthier eating patterns, or have factors such as reduced leisure time and the financial crisis increased consumption of packaged and processed foods?

I believe that one of the "good" effects of the financial crisis is that, as the Modern Greek person felt that he no longer had "control" over many issues related to his life, he turned his attention to taking control of his diet, to the extent that he was able to afford, believing (wrongly or not) that he will be in more complete charge of his life, health, work, etc. Many correctly turn to local produce from rural areas, but many others fall victim to the misinformation and general exaggeration that is prevalent regarding nutrition and are more likely to resort to orthorexia. So, while most people start exercising and eating their daily meals - as Greeks will have their occasional lamb chop - on the one hand, we have mountain tea and eggs from the farm and on the other, quinoa and salmon from America. Indeed, the Greek land grows nutritional treasures; turmeric is in no way superior to Saffron from Kozani nor goji berries are better than the raisins.

What should we pay special attention to in labels of food we consume daily for anyone trying to make healthier choices in their purchases?

In simple terms: Each of us should be able to distinguish most of the ingredients listed on a food label. For example, don't you find it odd that "wood rosin" is included in juice or "calcium sorbate" in a baked doe product? The best-case scenario would be anything we eat being as close to natural or otherwise homemade. The more E, pigment, and artificial sweeteners we find on a label, the less frequently we and our children (especially our children) should consume this product. Let's try to choose wholegrain products with reduced sugar and salt content and prefer products with honey, black sugar, and natural, unprocessed salt. Mind that every processed product we consume, even those processed by ourselves, is accompanied by fresh food, fruit or vegetables, thus enhancing our body's antioxidant capacity. Because nowadays finding "safe food" can be a difficult, or even a harrowing and expensive undertaking, let's try our best to buy it from "organic" food stores, especially children's daily milk - and we should be careful even there: It is best to have someone we know and trust, who will supply us with vegetables and fruit from their garden. The same goes for oil, meat and eggs and ideally for cheese or yoghurt. Even in big cities such as Athens or Thessaloniki, there are shops in every neighbourhood that bring local produce from the provinces daily, with the producer's signature, who comes from there and loves his place. So, let's become our best friend. Lastly, it would be best to have variety in our diet since the greater the variety of foods we consume weekly, the less the amount of a particular type of food we will eventually be eating, and the less likely it is for something to happen to us - e.g., addiction or infection from the concentration of some ingredient in a food or infectious or aggravating factor in our body. But this way we get a lot more nutrients and our taste buds are more satisfied.

9.1.2 Interview of Dietitian-Nutritionist Evangelos Zoumbaneas for "Provocateur.gr" Portal by Vicky Kalofotia, August 2014

"Orthorexia": An eating disorder, or a "disease" turned into a scourge?

We knew that in the case of people who have diet obsession symptoms, reaching and often exceeding the limits of starvation, we exclusively face, according to experts, with the disease called "anorexia", which in extreme cases can even lead to death.

However, as revealed by the relevant literature and daily clinical practice, there is another similar "disease" that has not yet been officially recognized despite having been identified since 1997.

> *'Orthorhexia' or otherwise "abnormal, extreme and excessive occupation with 'healthy' eating and consuming biologic 'clean food' and avoiding foods that are considered 'unhealthy' resulting in the creation of many dietary restrictions" says dietitian-Nutritionist and Managing Director of the Centre for Education and Treatment of Eating Disorders (CETED), Mr. Evangelos Zoumbaneas.*

"In orthorexia, the patients initially want to improve their health to cure a disease or lose weight, and eventually diet becomes the most important part of their lives," Mr. Zoumbaneas continued, adding that "the manifestation of this eating disorder appears to be more common in men than in women, as well as in people with lower levels of education."

Also, "it is no coincidence that because of the crisis - financial and not – more and more people are turning to healthy eating, unable to cope with the uncertainty of tomorrow, to feel in control."

And why has it not been officially recognized as a disease so far?

"Because clear distinction criteria for orthorexia have not yet been established, apart from in extreme cases, and there is debate as to whether it belongs to the group of eating disorders or so-called obsessive-compulsive disorders. Soon, however, it seems it will officially be recognized.

At present, however, it is already being used as a diagnosis by some health professionals who have documented the catastrophic effects of this condition", states Mr Zoumbaneas, and we immediately wonder about the rate at which "orthorexia" manifests in our country.

"Just because psychogenic orthorexia is not included in the Diagnostic Manual of Mental Disorders and therefore does not officially exist as a disease, there is no data for its exact definition, diagnostic criteria and occurrence rates, both in Greece and worldwide.

However, the average prevalence rate of orthorexia was 6.9% for the general population and 35-57.8% for high-risk groups such as health professionals and artists."

As the conversation went on, I remembered that during my internet research on orthorexia, I was often confronted with its association with anorexia nervosa, which is also a disease whose frequency rates have soared dramatically.

Are there really commonalities between these two eating disorders?

"In both, food plays a major role in the lives and relationships of inflicted people, due to social problems, personal need for control, compulsion or obsession, and perfection.

In anorexia nervosa and orthorexia, individuals have significant dietary restrictions and food stereotypes while living on a strict diet plan with many regulations experiencing high stress and stress to adhere to, without exception.

They also feel guilty and remorseful when they have not eaten as they had wanted or even when they have not exercised as much as they would have liked, since often the element of excessive exercise coexists."

Finally, we asked Mr. Zoumbaneas if there is any cure for treating or alleviating the symptoms and consequences of "orthorexia" in the human body.

"Moderation is the key to all areas of our lives. Because the person with orthorexia does not feel that he has a problem and believes that he knows everything about proper nutrition, he must realize the problem and get the appropriate information from a specialised dietitian.

Psychotherapy would also help the person discover what caused this obsession, resolve possible underlying emotional issues, and become more flexible and less dogmatic regarding eating. Therefore, a professional, specialised in the treatment of eating disorders is the best option."

9.2 Key Takeaways

1. **The complexity of orthorexia:**
    - Orthorexia is an obsession with eating "pure" and "healthy" foods, which can lead to excessive restrictions and harm both physical and mental health.
    - It's not officially classified as an eating disorder but shares characteristics with OCD and other disordered eating patterns.
2. **Understanding the symptoms:**
    - Look out for signs like extreme focus on food quality, guilt over "impure" foods, and avoidance of social situations involving food.
    - Recognizing these behaviours is the first step toward addressing them.
3. **The risks of rigid thinking:**
    - Overly strict food rules can disrupt your overall well-being, causing nutritional deficiencies and social isolation.
    - Flexibility and balance are essential in any healthy diet.
4. **The importance of professional guidance:**
    - Trained dietitians and mental health professionals can help you develop a more balanced relationship with food.
    - Seeking support is a strength, not a weakness.
5. **Reframe your approach to health:**
    - Focus on how food makes you feel rather than labeling foods as "good" or "bad."
    - A balanced and mindful approach to eating promotes long-term health and happiness.

6. **Build self-awareness:**
    - Reflect on your eating habits and the motivations behind them.
    - Self-awareness can help you identify and challenge unhelpful thoughts or behaviors.
7. **Celebrate flexibility:**
    - Allow yourself to enjoy a wide variety of foods without guilt.
    - Embrace moderation as the key to sustainable and enjoyable eating habits.

Chapter 10

Basic Guidelines for Nutrition Organisation

Each question can be expressed in two different ways. You either want to or you don't...

10.1 Basic Guidelines to Organise Daily Nutrition

10.1.1 Basic Instructions to Organise Our Daily Nutrition

An essential requirement for uplifting your body, in combination with the proper nutrition suggested later in this chapter, is sufficient rest that will be achieved with at least six hours of continuous night-time sleep. Before each meal, always drink a glass of water; during the meal, drink a cup of green tea or other beverages that significantly aid digestion and act as a diuretic, following liquid retention by the body.

During the day, you can eat the following snacks:

A tablespoon of **raw, unsalted nuts** such as walnuts, pecan walnuts, raw, unsalted almonds, cashews, macadamia, pistachios, Brazilian walnuts, etc. which you should first have soaked in water for 30-60 minutes.

Nutritional Intelligence: The Answer to Bulimia, Overeating, and Obesity
Evangelos Zoumbaneas

ISBN 978-981-5129-74-8 (Hardcover), 978-981-5129-73-1 (Paperback), 978-1-003-65188-8 (eBook)
www.jennystanford.com

A good idea is to soak them with a spoonful of dried fruit such as raisins, dried cherries, oatmeal, blackberries, or two dried figs or plums. You can pour the water into a pot that you want to fertilize. You may also prepare larger quantities and store in the refrigerator.

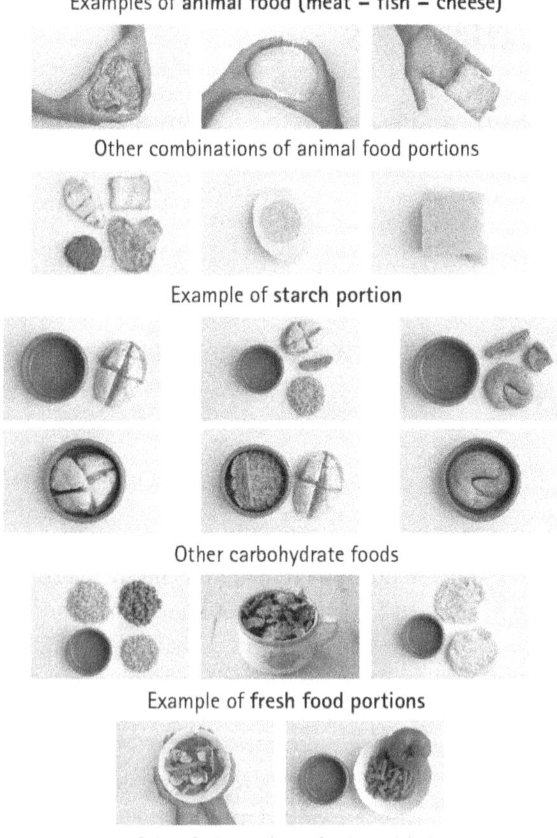

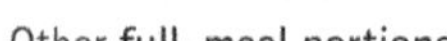

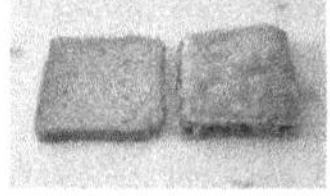

Figure 10.1 Quantities and portions.

This way, you will achieve the maximum intake of nutrients and beneficial fats from the fruits. The softer fibre will allow for better deconstruction and absorption of the nutrients from the body.

Other snacks you can use are:

Two **small digestive biscuits with no sugar**.

Half of a **small wholegrain bun**.

A **bar of Honey Oatmeal** from honey-oat-tahini.

Or two **wholegrain crackers** or two small rusks.

A wide **variety of nuts and dried fruit** and many other healthy snacks in balanced combinations can also be found in the online store: www.drplus.gr as they were chosen and compiled by Evangelos Zoumbaneas.

Drink mountain tea or green tea with each meal and preferably accompany your dinner with chamomile.

An essential prerequisite for any diet program's success is to accompany it with physical activity such as exercising, walking, etc., for at least for 30 minutes, five to six times a week.

10.1.2 What Is a Serving of Food?

Using the methods described in more detail in the book *THIN... Positive: Secrets to Control Hunger and Nutrition*, we will guide you on exactly how to eat and understand how much food you need without help.

The optimal way to do this is to organize your meals in at least three triples and two intermediate pairs to help you get a "personal regulator" of appetite and satiety.

But for some foods, such as meat, fish or cheese, it would be useful to have a sense of the quantity we need. Because we consider food weighing an unnecessarily strict method, we will give you a way to calculate servings based on your body. For example, if we were to serve pork stakes to a 1.85 tall man and a 1.60 tall woman, we can safely assume that we would choose a larger one for the former and a smaller one for the latter. A practical way to calculate servings based on our physique is: To calculate a portion of meat, we form a circle with both our palms' thumbs and index fingers. The circle formed, about the thickness of the index finger, is about the size of a medium boneless steak. This is also the volume of two or three small burgers or a small or large chicken breast, always depending on each person's fingers' size. In the same way, we can calculate the amount of a serving of fish. Only this time we will use the larger circle formed by our thumbs and middle fingers instead index fingers. Imagine this size as a fish without its head or tail, or a perch, swordfish or salmon fillet. Simply put, because fish has much less fat than red meat does, we can always eat a little more. We can calculate our serving of cheese using a different finger formation. If we bring our index, middle and ring finger together, from the base of the fingers to the top, a rectangular shape is formed, the volume of which is our individual cheese serving. If the cheese contains more fat, we calculate the serving based on the volume occupied by the index and middle finger. And that's because the harder a cheese is, the more fat it contains.

The size of a potato, when mentioned, will be considered as occupying the volume of a tennis ball. The amount of "a cup" will refer to the same volume as an individual yoghurt container, weighing 200-220 g. All other quantities will be measured in teaspoons or tablespoons.

SHOPPING LIST:

- Medium sized flatbreads or tortillas (preferably made with wholegrain flour)
- Wholemeal or Zeas flour bread (sourdough)
- Barley rusks, small sized - 40 gr, and medium sized - 60 gr
- Fresh fruit
- Fresh vegetables (lettuce, cabbage, carrots, peppers, spinach, broccoli, cauliflower, etc.)
- Frozen vegetables (green beans, peas)
- Pre-made salads
- Dried nuts
- Dried fruit
- Tahini - peanut butter
- Honey
- Vegetable milk (almond or soy, or coconut)
- Cheese
- Yoghurt
- Kefir
- Legumes

- Fresh or frozen corn
- Brown rice

10.1.3 How to Have Proper Meals

Our body is a perfect machine, which is tuned to work correctly even in conditions of food-shortage, to keep us alive. However, this ideal setup for our survival comes at odds with today's society of abundance, often leading us to over-eating. Of course, all this would serve the primitive man to store the energy needed to survive, even in adverse conditions. However today, even in "adverse conditions", or when we are stressed, we still have access to food - in particular, the harsher the circumstances, the more calorie-laden the food we crave is. This is why we continue to store fat without using it. That is why we need to adjust our satiety mechanism with clever tricks to teach our bodies to be satiated with the proper servings.

It is crucial to remember the "magic twenty-minute time frame". The human body cannot realize whether it has been satiated before twenty minutes have passed form the beginning of the meal, no matter how much food we have consumed. It is not a perfect computer that we provide with input, press a button and get a result. From the moment the first bite enters the mouth, touching the sublingual capillaries, the body begins to perceive the input of food. Still, to ensure our survival, the message of satiety has been programmed to reach the brain along with the rise in blood glucose levels, the synthesis of neurotransmitters and neuropeptides and serotonin, which is after twenty minutes have passed.

Because of this mechanism, we should only serve one serving, proper for our body and needs, chew our food well (at least 10 times), and give our body time to enjoy this process, the tastes, textures and smells. If we are hungry after twenty minutes, then the body really needs more food.

There are some tricks to help our body get full.

- Consuming a glass of water of fresh juice about 20-30 minutes before a meal and having a cup of tea or other digestive beverage with our food is very beneficial. We will continue drinking after the meal is over.

- As a first dish, we can have a warm or cold, light vegetable soup, low in calories, with no cream and fat to cover our stomach volume. Also, a cup of meat broth helps to eat less and enhances good gastrointestinal health. We could also use ready-made organic soups with glutamine monosodium.
- Before starting our meal, we can also eat half an apple and the other half after the meal, thus signalling the end of food ingestion and assisting its digestion. The same can be done with another fruit or with some yogurt or a glass of kefir.
- Other tools for signalling the end of a meal could be a cup of coffee, tea or cocoa beans, chewing gum or candy, or even a spoonful of nuts with little honey or dried fruit.
- Finally, one method that helps to signal the end of a meal is tooth brushing: Brushing off the meal removes any food residue. This is how the brain is instructed that our meal is over.

10.1.4 Diet and Its Secrets for Controlling Hunger and Satiety

For those who have tried every "diet" in the market, the prospect of learning to eat properly, minding the hunger and satiety mechanisms again, is a great challenge. Another significant point is remaining in good spirit while you are on a diet, watching your body improving day by day, observing changes in your clothes, and learning to take care of yourself without depending on the weighing scales. Providing yourself what you need and not much more. Aiming at taking care of ourselves, our health improves, our self-esteem increases, along with our self-image, we experience delayed ageing, while our body regaining its ideal weight is but a mere "side-effect" of this restorative process.

For this to happen, we need to ensure two things: 1) the proper production of serotonin by our body throughout the day and 2) the balance of glucose in our blood. Serotonin, the hormone of joy, boosts positive mood - which is why most antidepressants artificially increase its concentration in the brain - and conveys three messages:

1. I'm OK.
2. I got it under control.
3. I have had ENOUGH.

To produce serotonin, our body's complex mechanisms require every major meal (breakfast, lunch, and dinner) to contain: (a) a serving of fresh food, e.g. a cup of fresh fruit or vegetable, or 1-2 tablespoons of dried fruit or juice, mainly for vitamin C; b) a serving of protein food, e.g. three fingers of soft cheese or two fingers of hard cheese, yoghurt, egg, one palm of meat or fish, seafood etc. for amino acids and especially tryptophan; and (c) a serving of starch, preferably whole grain, e.g. a potato soup, rice, legumes, corn, pasta, etc. for carbohydrates, fibre, magnesium and B complex vitamins. One of the main meals should be lighter, e.g., salad with chicken and rusk or yoghurt with nuts and fruit.

Provided that the serotonin produced requires a "magic twenty-minute time frame" to act, we need to eat slowly, chewing well so that each meal lasts at least 20 minutes. After twenty minutes, we can see whether we have had enough. If not, one or two tablespoons of nuts or dried fruit can save us! Serotonin levels in the brain drop slowly after eight hours, so at most every eight hours, we need to renew the triad to produce serotonin again and maintain its positive effect throughout our day.

As for glucose, we must remember that after 3-3.5 hours of fasting or after one hour of exercise, blood levels fall below 0.8 mg, causing slight hypoglycaemia, which wakes up a "beast" in our body. This has a negative effect on our mood, concentration, causes nervousness or drowsiness and a feeling of fatigue. When stress levels fall, and we regain access to food, we eat uncontrollably. If we consume foods rich in simple sugars, with no nutritional value, e.g., chocolate, we can't stop – we wake up another beast - and we're even more hungry.

That is why no one can eat just one sweet. If one has been on an empty stomach since breakfast (e.g. at 9 am) having eaten nothing all day (only coffee, cigarettes or fast food), then at 9 pm he will have four beasts to satisfy and is very likely to consume food for all four of them at once. We can weaken hypoglycaemic beasts smartly by feeding them a proper source of glucose, such as fresh fruit, along with some snacks high in fibre, e.g., soaked nuts, cereal bars or nuts and cereal bars, etc., to avoid reactive hypoglycaemia and feel satiated for longer.

We should not forget to drink 10 glasses of water as, for each glass, our metabolism works at -10% and not miss opportunities for bitter or sour flavours that boost our metabolism (e.g., black coffee, bitter greens, lemon etc.). When we want something extra, e.g., sweet, we eat normally, before and after and preferably consume it with or even better after nutritious, e.g., fruit and nuts, and then the sweet.

Finally, physical activity is indispensable in all its forms that are possible and pleasurable (walking, yoga, fitness, dancing, etc.), enhancing our good mood with the produced "endorphins" and giving up to a 60 % of the success of a diet program, as "the loss of extra body fat is a matter of athletic time".

10.1.5 Ideas for 3-Course Meal Combinations

10.1.5.1 Triads for breakfast

- oatmeal porridge and chopped fruit
- two tablespoons of tahini or peanut butter with one fresh fruit and one glass of almond milk
- milk with two small oat biscuits and one fruit
- yoghurt with oats, honey and raisins
- yoghurt with oat jam and ground dried nuts
- toast with cottage cheese, jam, dried nuts, fruit
- toast with tahini, honey, fruit, dried nuts and a glass of almond milk or kefir
- a slice of bread, an egg and a glass of juice
- cherry tomatoes with cheese and a rusk
- baked nutmeg and fruit
- almond milk with oat honey and raisins
- smoothie with banana, kefir, oats, honey and cocoa

10.1.5.2 Triads for lunch with legumes

All legumes are combined with a serving of animal food such as cheese or a small serving of fish and can be accompanied with five large or ten small olives and a fresh salad.

- black-eyed peas with spinach
- black-eyed peas with tuna made in a pot
- chickpea soup
- chickpeas with red pepper and mushrooms
- baked chickpeas with onions and carrots
- falafel made with chickpeas
- grilled beans with turkey

- bean soup
- lentil soup
- peas made in the pot with a little potato

10.1.5.3 Triad for lunch with cooked vegetables

Cooked vegetables are combined with a serving of protein such as cheese or a small serving of fish and a moderate nut or a two-slice bread or wholegrain breadcrumbs and a fresh salad.

- mushroom fricassee
- grilled mushrooms with gruyere
- mushroom soup
- mushrooms stuffed with minced meat
- beans
- baked okra
- green celery with rice
- cabbage with rice
- vegetarian burger
- vegetable risotto with feta cheese
- stuffed vegetables with rice
- eggplants stuffed with rice, onions, tomato
- omelette with vegetables
- spinach with rice
- eggplant with potatoes made in a pot
- baked potatoes
- cannelloni stuffed with minced eggplants

10.1.5.4 Triad for minced meat

They are almost always combined with a fresh salad and a medium sized rusk or two thin slices of bread or a cup of potato or rice or corn or other cooked starch.

- Cabbage rolls with lemon sauce
- meatballs with rice boiled in a lemony broth (Greek dish called “Giouvarlakia”)
- mince roll in the oven with roasted vegetables
- light pasticcio
- pasta with minced meat or spaghetti
- mushrooms stuffed with minced meat
- aubergines stuffed with minced meat or mozzarella or gruyere

- meatballs made in a saucepan with lemon, carrots, potatoes, mustard
- grilled burgers with sauce and rice
- burger with potato salad

10.1.5.5 Triads for dinner

- tortilla with roasted vegetables Philadelphia, ham, turkey
- oatmeal porridge
- milk, oats, honey and raisins
- potato salad, feta cheese, tomatoes and olives
- potherb with a serving of cheese and a medium sized rusk
- egg, salad, cherry tomatoes and rusk
- sandwiches with gouda, ham, mustard, tomato, mushrooms
- sandwiches with cream cheese, salmon and lettuce
- egg sandwich with cucumber, tomato, light mayonnaise
- pitta-based pizza
- tuna salad with tomato, cucumber, carrot, rusk
- tuna salad with lettuce, dill, light mayonnaise, cucumber
- skewer with tomato, pitta baked without oil and yoghurt
- Pitta, salad, meat skewers
- Greek salad with tomato, feta cheese, cucumber and rusks
- rusks with cottage cheese, turkey and tomato
- trahana with feta cheese and cucumber
- roasted eggs with chopped tomatoes and a slice of toasted bread
- egg tortilla, yoghurt, pickles, mustard, grated carrot
- chef salad with lettuce, cherry tomatoes, cucumber, egg, ham, gouda and a little sauce

10.1.5.6 Online information for your meal planning

More on "Hunger and Nutrition Control Secrets" can be found in the book *THIN... Positive* by Evangelos Zoumbaneas by "KEADD" Publications, https://amzn.to/46HrnF9.
The Spanish language edition of the book *THIN... POSITIVE, SECRETOS PARA CONTROLAR EL HAMBRE Y LA DIETA* is available at https://www.amazon.com/Thin-Positive-SECRETOS-CONTROLAR-Spanish-ebook/dp/B0842XJBSS/ref=sr_1_1?crid=3J3QAXY90A7EM&dib=eyJ2IjoiMSJ9.UbYBGxI1TY-9IAuFi0UHKQ.tBAXqpW2-O_2GzDGhYD2KB2YYJGI1KUNlXKUW6yeNWM&dib_tag=se&keywords=

THIN...+positive+SECRETOS+PARA+CONTROLAR+EL+HAMBRE+Y+LA+DIETA&qid=1742807216&s=digital-text&sprefix=thin...+positive+secretos+para+controlar+el+hambre+y+la+dieta%2Cdigital-text%2C423&sr=1-1.

Ideas for easy combinations organized in triads and smart snacks are available at www.diatrofi.gr.

If you are on Instagram, check and add your own triads with hashtag #3adadiatrofi and check for more ideas in the hashtag #diatrofigr & #zoumbaneas.e.

For better information, Like our page on Facebook: diatrofi.gr.

For the Professional Training Courses in Eating Disorders & Nutrition) please visit the website: www.eating-disorders.org.uk

For the Professional Training Courses in Eating Disorders & Nutrition) in Greek Language, please visit the website: www.keadd.gr.

If you want to communicate with a Greek Speaker specialist in eating disorders, please visit https://diet-coaching.gr/en/.

You can find a wide range of useful products for your diet on the site www.drplus.gr by Evangelos Zoumbaneas, such as recipes online and all the books of the Eating Disorders Training Centre with 5% discount for every purchase, using the discount coupon code: PLUS100. Alternatively, call +30 210 2718542, and provide your discount code.

10.2 A Healthy Intestine as the Basis for Happiness

10.2.1 Connection of the Intestine with the Central Nervous System

The two-way communication between the central nervous system and the gut microbiome has been the object of great interest in recent years. The gastrointestinal tract connects to the brain via a vital nerve called the pulmonary gastric nerve. It resembles a cable that connects the heart, gastrointestinal tract, and lungs to the brain. It is connected to the area of the brain called the hypothalamus, which controls emotions and various functions such as hunger and thirst.

10.2.2 What Is the Intestinal Microbiome?

The intestinal microbiome is a vast ecosystem of organisms that includes bacteria, fungi, viruses and protozoa that live in our digestive tracts and weigh about 2 kg (heavier than the average brain). Modern medicine now considers the intestinal microbiome as a separate organ of the human body. Dysbiosis (that is, the imbalance between "good" and "bad" intestinal flora) and intestinal inflammation have been linked to several mental illnesses, including anxiety and depression, prevalent in society today. Proper probiotics can restore normal microbial balance and therefore play a role in the treatment and prevention of anxiety and depression.

Healthy bowel function has been linked to the normal function of the central nervous system (CNS). It is known that the hormones, neurotransmitters and immune agents released from the intestine send signals to the brain either directly or via autonomous neurons.

It is becoming apparent that the gut and brain axis extends even beyond these two systems, as in endocrine, neural and immune pathways.

Recently, studies have surfaced, that focus on changes in the gut microbiome and the effect of these change on various central nervous system (CNS) disorders, including, but not limited to anxiety, depressive disorders, schizophrenia and autism.

10.2.3 Additional Ways of Communication between Bowel and Brain

The intestine and the brain are also linked through chemicals called neurotransmitters.

For example, the neurotransmitter called serotonin contributes to feelings of happiness, satiation and pleasure.

Interestingly, 80% of these neurotransmitters are also produced by the intestinal cells and the trillions of microbes. Much of the serotonin, endorphins and dopamine is made in the gut.

The gut microbes also produce the neurotransmitter called γ-aminobutyric acid (GABA) and help control feelings of fear and anxiety.

Studies in laboratory mice have shown that certain probiotics can increase the neurotransmitter OBAA and reduce depression-like stress and behaviour.

10.2.4 How Does the Intestine Relate to Daily Life Stress?

The hypothalamus controls emotions but also executes another critical function: the regulation of stress. Stress is the body's response to something happening in our environment. Examples of daily stressful activities are almost all day-to-day activities such as exercising through sports, preparing for an impending school exam, or completing all the necessary tasks on time during work. In the human body, the nervous system and the hypothalamic-pituitary-adrenal

(HPA) axis, which connects the nervous system and the endocrine system, are the central systems that respond to stress.

The microbiome-gut-brain (MGB) axis is a two-way link between the gut bacteria and the brain. It links the nervous, endocrine, and immune systems; it resembles a direct telephone line between the gut bacteria and the brain. The MOB axis is a neuroendocrine-immune system. This means that it connects the nervous system, the endocrine system and the immune system.

The hypothalamic-pituitary-adrenal (HPA) axis is comprised of glands that produce a cortisol hormone and prepares the body to deal with stressful conditions. This hormone indicates to the body cells that must produce energy to cope with a stressful situation, by increasing the level of blood sugar, suppressing the immune system that protects the body from diseases, and promoting the mobilization of fats and proteins. The presence of bacteria helps us have a stronger immune system that learns from them how to protect the body from various diseases. When the body comes in contact with bacteria, it increases its defences. Improved defence reduces bad bacteria and improves the environment for good bacteria, turning the gastrointestinal tract into an ideal environment for them.

10.2.5 Stress Changes the Intestinal Flora

Some environmental conditions that cause us great anxiety or make us feel sad can cause a stress response in the body that may last for weeks, months or even years.

This long-term stress can alter the normal function of the hypothalamic-pituitary- adrenal (HPA) axis. This means that the human body may experience problems with its stress response after a prolonged stressful situation.

Long-term stress can harm the bacteria in the gut. This is because the hypothalamic- pituitary-adrenal (HPA) axis is also associated with the microbiome-gut- brain (MGB) axis. Since communication via the axis can occur in any direction, stress factors that affect the brain can also damage the intestine and the bacteria living inside.

A difficult situation in a person's daily life can be enough to reduce the diversity (the number of different species) of gut bacteria and increase the number of bad bacteria in the area. These changes in the gut microbes can, in turn cause changes in the function of the brain.

The brain is part of the nervous system and, being the centre for operations of the body, it orders our muscles to move, and interprets all the things we feel and live.

10.2.6 What Is Depression, and How Does It Appear?

Depression is a brain disorder that affects emotions. People with depression feel sad and guilty for a long period of time. However, we do not know the exact mechanism that causes it. Changes in the body that lead to the development of the disease are likely to involve the three systems that form the microbiome-gut-brain axis. The nervous, endocrine and immune systems, along with emotional stress, malnutrition and high use of antibiotics, are risk factors that can alter the microbiome-gut-brain axis, increasing the risk of its appearance.

The best "dowry" for a child's health is a robust microbiome.

The microbiome of every human being begins to exist from the first day of its existence, given as a "dowry" through regular childbirth.

But there is one crucial distinction that can significantly influence many factors in the baby's future health. This distinction is that infants born naturally (vaginally) had more significant amounts of bacteria in their intestine than infants born by caesarean section.

From the very first week of life, the gastrointestinal colonization of microbial flora is extremely dynamic. This crucial period during creation and development of the microbiome is essential for a newborn's health and immunity. During this period, the underdevelopment of germs has been associated with numerous conditions, such as stress, septicaemia, cardiovascular disease, and atopic disease.

10.2.7 Difference between Breastfeeding and Packaged Foods in Infant Gut Microbiome

Early nutrition is also very important, which appears to play an essential role in shaping the growing microbial gut flora.

Breastfeeding is directly related to immunity of the intestines and mucus membranes. One of the most important effects of breast-feeding is that it reduces the levels of certain toxic substances (pro-inflammatory cytokines) that generally cause acute and chronic inflammation. Breastfeeding also reduces the chance of gastroenteritis.

A recent study found that infants fed with dietary formulas during the first four weeks had a significantly reduced total bacterial species population, compared to breast milk that provides a variety of oligosaccharides, including lactose, different non-digestible molecules (non-digestible sugars) which are also the main food for the development of good intestinal flora and the maintenance of bacterial strains.

10.2.8 Effects of Microbial Flora on the Body

Dietary alterations can have a significant effect on bacterial intestinal composition in as little as 24 hours. However, the bacterial composition is restored if the change in diet is only temporary. Regardless of the species endemic to the gut, as long as their symbiotic role (when living in harmony) is the same, their host will live normally and without health problems. Symbiotic bacteria help:

- In the proper function of the immune system
- In intestinal homoeostasis
- Good amino acid metabolism
- The destruction of toxins
- In the excellent production and absorption of vitamins
- Digestion of macronutrients (proteins, carbohydrates, fats)

Bacteria can convert food into energy for the human body. In fact, of all the foods consumed by the gut, gut bacteria utilize about 10% of the energy that will then be used by the body throughout the day.

10.2.9 An Adult's Microbiome

Due to many factors such as diet, environment, season and health status of a person, it is almost impossible to define a "normal" microbiome.

When the human microbiome is threatened through diet, stress or antibiotics, the normal microflora undergoes changes. A dysbiosis leads to increased intestinal permeability, destroys the inner wall that isolates the intestine from the rest of the body, and allows contents such as bacterial metabolites, molecules, and the bacteria themselves to leak into the bloodstream, a phenomenon that is accurately called "leaky" or permeable bowel syndrome. "

Increased intestinal permeability leads to harmful effects on the immune system and diseases such as inflammatory bowel disease (IBD), diabetes, asthma and psychiatric disorders, including depression, anxiety and autism.

10.2.10 Intestinal Inflammation and Psychology

An inflammation of the gastrointestinal tract can cause microbial stress in the gut which causes the release of cytokines and neurotransmitters. The former are proteins secreted by cells of the immune system when they encounter a pathogenic microorganism or other potential danger, activating other immune cells, thereby increasing the body's defence. Coupled with increased intestinal permeability, these molecules systematically travel in the bloodstream while they should not be there in the first place. Their passage through the intestine into the bloodstream causes problems, increasing the permeability of the blood-brain barrier. Their release affects the brain's function, leading to anxiety, depression and memory loss.

The disease probably starts primarily when cytokine release takes place and secondarily due to an overly strong response to stressors in the body. It is now known that pro-inflammatory cytokines play a role in the development of anxiety and depression associated with a state of chronic inflammation. Pro-inflammatory cytokines also stimulate the hypothalamic-pituitary-adrenal axis and eventually lead to cortisol production via the adrenal glands. This known stress hormone works negatively in this case.

10.2.11 Prebiotics and Psychology

An examination of the effects of prebiotics on mood, performed at the University of Oxford's Department of Psychiatry, yielded promising results.

Prebiotics are complex carbohydrates that humans cannot digest but are the essential food for probiotic bacteria. Essentially, prebiotics are dietary fibres that nourish the bacteria we already have in our gut.

So, our diet is probably the most important route for maintaining a healthy axis between the gut and the brain. A balanced diet, including, among others, fish, vegetables, cereals, fruits, nuts soaked in water, fermented milk products such as traditional yoghurt, kefir, sour milk, cheese (when consumed uncooked), and water, can achieve it. The food we eat has a direct impact on our bacteria and their home - our bodies.

Patients suffering from depression benefit from maintaining a healthy and balanced diet by providing proper nutrition to preservation of their gut microbiome.

Prebiotics are unlikely to replace medicine used to treat mental illness. Still, they could aid in the better function of these medicine for people who do not respond well.

10.2.12 Probiotics for the Treatment of Intestine and Mood

In patients with inflammatory bowel disease, probiotics were associated with fewer cytokines and improved intestinal permeability. The administration of probiotics also led to a reduction in inflammation.

Probiotics have a neuroprotective role as they prevent stress from causing neuronal dysfunction.

Studies in humans and animals on probiotics, show a decrease in anxiety and depressive symptoms. Specifically, in a 30-day study, healthy volunteers with no prior depression symptoms were homogenously divided into two groups. The first one received probiotics and the second one antidepressant medicine. Subjects who had received probiotics showed decreased cortisol levels and improved self-reported psychological effects, similar to the individuals who had received anxiolytic.

When comparing the probiotics with the antidepressant escitalopram in mice, the probiotics proved to have similar results. Probiotics have had the same success in reducing stress and have been more effective than the antidepressant for maintaining healthy metabolism and body weight. Oral ingestion of probiotics also resulted in an increase in tryptophan, a precursor to serotonin, which is the main hormone of joy.

Recent research has shown that the use of fermented foods in diets provides gastrointestinal and cognitive benefits.

Advantages of probiotics over other medication include ease of availability, lower cost, less dependency and fewer side effects. Regulation of the micro flora composition offers the potential to improve the intestinal immunity, homeostasis, and protection from inflammation.

However, until there is more evidence for use of probiotics as a treatment for anxiety and depressive disorders, probiotics in any form cannot be considered a reliable treatment compared to psychiatric medications.

Obesity, lifestyle, tobacco use, alcohol, ionizing radiation, stress, heavy metals, and antibiotics, either through oral or reckless use of animals and then consumed by people, may affect the overall benefits of probiotics.

10.2.13 Foods that Help the Microbiome-Gut-Brain (MGB) Axis

Omega-3 fatty acids: These fats are found in fatty fish (sardines, fresh salmon, anchovies, swordfish, sea bream, anchovies, red seaweed, etc.) and, in large quantities, in the human brain. Studies in humans and animals have shown that omega-3 fatty acids can increase the gut's "good" bacteria and reduce the risk of brain disorders.

Fermented foods: Yoghurt, kefir, cabbage, peas, sauerkraut, olives, kefir or sour milk, pickles (the pasteurization process neutralizes friendly bacteria; the best solution is to make your own pickles at home using just salt and water), miso, and ripe cheeses contain healthy germs such as lactic acid bacteria.

Foods rich in fibre: Wholegrain products, nuts, seeds, fruits and vegetables all contain prebiotic fibres that are beneficial for gut bacteria. Prebiotics (which are abundant in all vegetables and especially in foods such as leeks, celery, asparagus, endive, wild greens, common artichoke, chicory, walnuts, green bananas, garlic, onions, etc.) can reduce the stress hormone in humans.

Foods rich in polyphenols: Cocoa, green tea, olive oil and coffee contain polyphenols, which are phytochemicals consumed by the gut bacteria. Polyphenols increase the population of healthy gut bacteria and can improve cognitive function.

Tryptophan-rich foods: Tryptophan is an amino acid that converts to serotonin. Foods rich in tryptophan include turkey, eggs and cheese, avocado, nuts and more.

10.2.14 Are We What We Eat After All?

Most beneficial bacteria are found in the mucosa, where they meticulously "train" our immune system, protect the stomach and intestinal tracts, consume what we do not need and produce vitamins. If the beneficial bacteria exist in harmony with the harmful ones, they make us stronger; the beneficial ones take care of us and keep us healthy at all levels.

It is important to understand that food has a more significant impact on our body and does not function merely as a source of calories.

A notion was prevalent in the past according to which we are what we eat: "Let your medicine be your food and let your food be your medicine." The inspiration for this saying was the great doctor of ancient times, Hippocrates. Now we have come to realise that this is not precisely the case, but instead, it would be preferably replaced it with the following: "We are everything we eat and can absorb."

Instead of thinking about calories, think about the nutrition and impact the food intake can have on the intestinal microflora. The more raw and less processed foods we can consume in our daily lives, the more our bodies will be rewarded with better health, both physically and mentally.

(*The text was first published in the portal www.diatrofi.gr by nutritionist Vassileios Katsilas*)

10.2.15 References

Gut microbiota's effect on mental health: The gut-brain axis. *Clin Pract.* 2017 Sep 15;7(4):987

Daulatzai MA. Non-celiac gluten sensitivity triggers gut dysbiosis, neuroinflammation, gut-brain axis dysfunction, and vulnerability for dementia. *CNS Neurol Disord* 2015;14:110-31.

Zhou L, Foster J. Psychobiotics and the gut-brain axis: in the pursuit of happiness. *Neuropsych Dis Treat* 2015;715.

Belkaid Y, Hand T. Role of the microbiota in immunity and inflammation. *Cell* 2014;157:121-41

Neufeld KM, Kang N, Bienenstock J, Foster JA. Reduced anxiety-like behavior and central neurochemical change in germ-free mice. *Neurogastroent Motil* 2011;23:264, e119.

10.3 Do I Need Nutritional Supplements?

Excerpt from the interview of nutritionist Evangelos Zoumbaneas for fmvoice.gr portal, May 2019, by journalist Maria Bakopoulou.

(1) What has been the trend regarding nutritional supplements lately? Do dietitians recommend them, or do they insist on vitamins that one can get from food?

Answer: As I have mentioned in my book *THIN... Positive – Secrets of Controlling Hunger and Nutrition*, no one needs dietary supplements provided everything he eats comes directly from his or her garden, drinks spring water, breathes exclusively the, much richer in oxygen content, country fresh air, he is busy at least three to four hours a day with his garden, interacting with the Earth and nature and gazing at the endless blue instead of watching television.

(2) I read that there has been an increasing trend in the use of dietary supplements in recent years ... What do you think this is owed to?

Answer: Just as I have described the conditions under which, one can be fed on nature's generous products, all those who live in the unnatural urban environment, need to supplement their diet. Daily stress, bad sleep (and, especially, at inappropriate hours that do not include the fundamental period of 23.00-5.00, that is, the hours when the growth hormones are activated for cell repair and detoxification of the body), as well as the many fast-food meals compel us to cover food deficiencies with selected nutritional supplements.

(3) What about Greece? Do Greeks trust food supplements more than they used to? Why? Is there an increase in their rate of use we can refer to?

Answer: As we move away from natural foods, and especially immediate access to them - that is, the ability to eat an orange directly from the tree which, at the time, may contain 60mg of vitamin C but a month later, when it comes to our table, the same orange may not contain more than 10mg - as long as we live in the shade and our skin does not come in direct contact with the sun for at least 20 minutes daily, to produce the necessary vitamin D, as long as we consume even one serving of food made with white flour and sugar e.g., a piece of cake, chocolate, croissant, or sweet, the body will not only fail to receive the necessary B vitamins, but also be stripped of any existing ones; affecting thus our metabolism and causing food to be stored as fat. As long as we drink a glass of alcohol daily, the nervous system's valuable vitamin B12 will be destroyed. Although the list of negative effects is long, I need to make a final mention to the destruction of intestinal flora by the use of antibiotics in animals and animal products: These substances pass through the food chain into the bacterial flora of the gut and destroy healthy bacteria responsible for the proper metabolism of foods into energy and nutrients, as well as for the production of antibodies and neurotransmitters which are directly related to physical, mental and psychological health.

(4) Is there a risk related to their consumption? And if so, to what extent?

Answer: First, before anyone takes any dietary supplement, extensive nutritional and medical history should be recorded by either a physician or a professional nutritionist-nutritionist, in combination with haematological and biochemical tests that should additionally include the values of factor D3 (TH) 25 or total D, B12, folic acid, iron, ferritin, fasting insulin, glycosylated haemoglobin, thyroid control. The health professional should then prepare the appropriate nutrition plan and the necessary supplementary treatment to cover possible immediate rehabilitation needs.

Then, after the essential deficiencies have been restored and if the person has significantly improved their daily eating habits, introduced regular exercise at a frequency of at least 3 times a week and sufficiently improved sleeping hours, then to continue maintaining control of his health, he will need to take at regular intervals:

- A natural multivitamin to cover most deficiencies in nutrients due to debasement of food in large cities.
- A vitamin C supplement of at least 500 mg
- A supplement of probiotics for lasting health balance of the intestines and consequently, the proper function of the immune system as well as the improvement of mental and psychological health. When choosing probiotics, it is preferable to prefer probiotics stored in the refrigerator as this will ensure the product's freshness and effectiveness.
- An Ω3 fatty acid supplement if fish consumption is less frequent than twice per week.
- A vitamin D3 supplement (in combination with vitamin K2 and magnesium for proper absorption), for every day that we do not come in direct contact with the sun for at least 20 minutes on bare (not through glass) and provided that we do not swim immediately afterwards to avoid washing off the oily form of the vitamin on the skin. This also means that we should not use sunscreen in the summer with a grade of protection greater than 10 because the valuable vitamin D is not formed on the skin. Ideally, keep your blood vitamin D3 levels constant within 40-50 units.

But I must reiterate that nutritional supplements should always be recommended by a qualified health professional who is constantly informed of all new developments in research and nutritional medicine from many independent sources and of course, always with proper nutritional treatment and constant medical supervision.

(5) What has changed nowadays and supplements are considered suitable for consumption, not only by athletes and individuals who undergo intense training, but also children?

Answer: Athletes use nutritional supplements strictly on condition that they are recommended by a team nutritionist or a professional nutritionist and under no circumstances by the trainer or salesperson. Any other form of suggestion of any supplement by a non-specialist physician or nutritionist will certainly soon lead to a severe health problem.

Children living in cities and following their parents' bad eating habits clearly require the right nutritional supplements for their own needs. Children born by caesarean section need supplemental treatment with probiotics, because due to this procedure they will acquire a robust microbiome compared to a child born by regular birth at 3 years old, provided that there is a pet in the house and the child is in regular contact with nature.

Probiotics are also vital every time someone young or old, receives antibiotics because without them, the microbial gut flora may never be restored, with unhealthy consequences for the health and dramatically increasing the likelihood of some autoimmune disease.

Certainly, all babies born should receive vitamin D3 supplementation and have their vitamin D levels checked twice a year, at the end of October and the end of March, to decide whether to keep taking the vitamin or not.

In conclusion, for those who do not live, as I explained at the outset, in conditions providing total tranquillity and excellent nutrition quality, proper and appropriate nutritional supplements - always combined with adequate rest and regular exercise - can promote health to such an extent that they are likely never take medication for some of the so-called "diseases of modern Western culture" such as diabetes, hypertension and metabolic syndrome.

10.4 Key Takeaways

1. **Organize your nutrition:**
    - Create a daily plan that includes balanced meals with quality ingredients.
    - Focus on the quality and quantity of food, prioritizing natural and healthy options.
2. **The importance of a healthy gut:**
    - Your gut is your "second brain" and significantly affects your physical and mental health.
    - Support your gut health with foods rich in probiotics and prebiotics.
3. **The truth about dietary supplements:**
    - Supplements can be helpful but should never replace a balanced diet.
    - Consult with experts before adding supplements to your routine.
4. **The concept of nutritional consistency:**
    - You don't have to be perfect every day; aim for overall consistency in your eating habits.
    - Trust the small, steady improvements you make.
5. **Turn challenges into opportunities:**
    - Learn to recognize when you're veering off track and use it as an opportunity to reassess your strategy.
    - Failures are lessons, not setbacks.
6. **Self-awareness is key:**
    - Track what you eat, how you feel, and which habits help you stay on track.
    - Understanding your body and mind is the foundation for any positive change.
7. **The power of consistency:**
    - Maintain balance in your diet and daily routine, regardless of circumstances.
    - Consistency is the cornerstone of lasting health and well-being.
    - These points can serve as a guide to help you organize your life and nutrition in a sustainable, meaningful, and balanced way.

Index

Get Professional Help

Get acquainted with our services and the Nutritional Intelligence therapeutic program at https://diet-coaching.gr/en/.

The site dietcoachings.gr is a specialized platform which offers holistic support to individuals suffering from eating disorders such as emotional eating, binge eating, anorexia nervosa and bulimia nervosa. Our cross-scientific team consists of professional nutritionists, psychologists, and physical education professors, specialized in managing eating disorders.

We provide individualized support to people with eating disorders:

Emotional Eating

Do you often feel confused with your diet and uncomfortable with your body?

Has food become an obsession, and you don't know how to control your appetite?

Have you gone on too many unsuccessful diets only to gain more and more weight?

It's time to be introduced to a new way of dealing with weight, get help to establish a better balance and develop skills relative to food and physical activity.

Binge Eating

Do you feel that your hunger is uncontrollable?

Is your weight increasing day by day and you seem unable to do anything about it?

Is food the only pleasure left for you?

Now you can seek help to regain a healthy relationship with food.

Anorexia Nervosa

Do you feel you are in a continuous effort to lose weight, even if others tell you that you are already too thin?

Has food become an obsession and you find yourself counting calories in every single meal you have?

Do you hear a voice inside you, always telling you to lose more weight?

If your life is an ever-going diet, it is time to relieve yourself of this suffering.

Bulimia Nervosa

Do you often lose control of how much you eat?

Are you constantly trying to get rid of the extra calories in any way possible?

Do you feel trapped in a vicious circle of one failed diet after another?

Now is the time to rid yourself of the daily burden of dieting.

Help for Children and Adolescents

Do you feel that your child has an obsession with food, trains excessively and eats too little?

Do they isolate every time they eat and gradually exclude more and more kinds of food from their diet?

If your instinct tells you that there's something wrong with their health, now is the right time to seek professional support and get proper guidelines on how to help them.

Dietary Intelligence Plan

Learn about the Nutritional Intelligence Program.

Certified Professionals

Health experts certified by the Greek Centre of Education and Treatment for Eating Disorders.

The Greek Centre of Education and Treatment for Eating Disorders is a certified organization specialized in treating patients suffering from eating disorders, and training health experts on how to be optimally prepared and skilled in treating patients with eating disorders since 2010.

Patients' Testimonies

I learned all about food combinations, having small meals, proper breakfast and so much more with a hands-on approach. Above all, I stopped punishing or rewarding myself with food...

(Despina M.)

I feel the need to express my gratitude but also my admiration for your struggle to support those who face eating disorders...

(Maria K.)

I didn't even know I was acting this way because of my Binge Eating Disorder. Thank you for reintroducing me with myself and changing my life. *(George A.)*

Ask for Evaluation

Book an Initial Evaluation Session with a health expert now and get informed about all different ways of treatment.

During the Initial Session, an "evaluation of eating behaviour and the possibility of an eating disorder" will take place with the use of specialized psychometric tools.

You will get in a video call with a professional dietologist or psychologist, specialized in eating disorders. They will give you an initial evaluation regarding the extent of the problem according to the results of the psychometric tools. The time needed for this initial evaluation is about 50 minutes.

The health expert will evaluate your initial request and will suggest the proper team of experts for you to proceed with your treatment, if you wish to do so. You will be presented with a treatment proposal, including the aforementioned steps, adjusted to your individual needs and daily habits.

There is a Solution!

With the right guidance and the proper treatment approach, every individual with a disturbed relationship with food can gain invaluable treatment time and avoid wasting money on methods and practices that may not fit their own needs.

If you wish, you may ask for general instructions, in the form of electronic files. They will help you better understand the issue that concerns you as well as provide you with general guidelines about the treatment process.

Nutritional Education and Psychologic Support Program

The Nutritional Education and Psychologic Support program concerns people who suffer from an unhealthy relationship with food.

It is based on the best-selling book *Nutritional Intelligence: The Answer to Bulimia, Overeating and Obesity*, by Evangelos Zoumbaneas, and the methodologies taught in the "Master Practitioner in Eating Disorders" training course. It is applied exclusively by health experts certified as "Master Practitioner in Eating Disorders" and includes specific therapeutic stages.

It is exclusively applied by health professionals and Master Practitioners in Eating Disorders and involves specific treatment stages.

The first step in therapy is the evaluation of the individual's eating habits and investigation for the possible existence of an eating disorder.

Are you ready to speak with the person who will change your life?

Contact us and schedule a free evaluation of eating behaviour and the possibility of an eating disorder at dietcoachings.gr.

The platform works in collaboration with the Greek Centre of Education & Treatment for Eating Disorders (keadd.gr), which specializes in training nutrition and health professionals as well as monitoring eating disorder treatments since 2010.

For more information or to book an initial evaluation session, please visit dietcoachings.gr or write to secretary@keadd.gr.

For Product Safety Concerns and Information please contact our EU representative GPSR@taylorandfrancis.com
Taylor & Francis Verlag GmbH, Kaufingerstraße 24, 80331 München, Germany

www.ingramcontent.com/pod-product-compliance
Ingram Content Group UK Ltd.
Pitfield, Milton Keynes, MK11 3LW, UK
UKHW020955130825
461793UK00018B/391

* 9 7 8 9 8 1 5 1 2 9 7 3 1 *